Go Vegan?

Review of Science

Part 2

By Milos Pokimica

Medical Disclaimer

The information provided in this book is just personal opinion of the author and is not intended or implied to be a substitute for professional medical advice, diagnosis or treatment. The information provided in this book is for informational purposes only and are not intended to serve as a substitute for the consultation, diagnosis, and/or medical treatment of a qualified physician or healthcare provider.

NEVER DISREGARD PROFESSIONAL MEDICAL ADVICE OR DELAY SEEKING MEDICAL TREATMENT BECAUSE OF SOMETHING YOU HAVE READ ON OR ACCESSED THROUGH THIS BOOK. NEVER APPLY ANY LIFESTYLE CHANGES OR ANY CHANGES AT ALL AS A CONSEQUENCE OF SOMETHING YOU HAVE READ IN THIS BOOK BEFOR CONSULTING LICENCED MEDICAL PRACTITIONER.

In the event of a medical emergency, call a doctor or 911 immediately. This book does not recommend or endorse any specific groups, organizations, tests, physicians, products, procedures, opinions, or other information that may be mentioned inside. Reliance on any information provided by this book is solely at your own risk.

None of the individual contributors, author, nor anyone else connected to this book can take any responsibility for the results or consequences of any attempt to use or adopt any of the information presented inside.

Warning:

This book contains images (which may be unsuitable for children and upsetting to adults) and topics and discussions which some readers might find upsetting.

Table of Contents:

Food and drug industry

"Was the government to prescribe to us our medicine and diet, our bodies would be in such keeping as our souls are now."

— Thomas Jefferson

In modern medicine, profit is mostly made on sick people. Healthy individuals are not very lucrative. You can sell them supplements, but that market is not where the real money is laying. Nobody around you will have the interest to tell you the whole truth and keep you healthy except you. It is only your job and nobody else's. It is not the job of your doctor. He does not care about your health. He is going to stop listening to you in seconds after you started speaking. What he is going to do is to write the prescription, and if anything goes wrong, he is also considering how to protect himself from liability. That is his real job. Even if he wanted to spend time on you, he would have a hard time because the doctors themselves do not know what the truth is and actually have life expectancy that is much shorter than average. Furthermore, even if there is some real cure the intention will be to silence it. Just cancer treatment drugs made industry $107 billion worldwide in 2015 and are projected to exceed $150 billion by 2020. And that is without an endless chain of medical tests, operations, support therapies. That is a reality. Also if you are youthful and don't have any medical conditions the brainwashing machine will fill you with fears and insecurities. You will see beautiful people heavily photoshopped on every magazine filled with commercials. You will need cosmetics, supplements, surgery and other self-improving products to make you happy. Why? Because you want to be better than your competition and get a good looking woman or handsome husband. This is the way evolution is condition our brain to enforce the highest survival chance of our offspring and to ensure that even in the peacetime there is a constant struggle to be better than your current rival. The struggle is a constant trait. We are evolutionary conditioned to fear and hate so that we can improve and adapt and survive. High happiness and love have nothing to do with survival in ever-changing habitats. There is nothing wrong in self-improvement, but that mindset is also what will make many individuals that do not have adequate analytic skills into a cycle of self-destruction. More intelligent members of our society will manipulate their fears for profit and control. Judging by the legislation that WHO is pushing and the industry standards for preventive medicine which is another scam the goal of public health policy in 21 century would be to spread constant fear for the ever larger and larger segment of the population. This might be hard to understand logically so I will rephrase it in this way.

Do you have any anxiety if you don't have health insurance? How about something insignificant like a dental plan? Do you have a fear if you do not check your self annually? What about that breast cancer or some other cancer prevention screening? Do you think that you would feel any anxiety if the doctor tells you that you have cancer? Do you believe that you would be able to live in constant fear of getting it if you have a genetic predisposition? Do you fear to disobey your doctor? What if you don't vaccinate your kids? It is mandatory. You do not even have a choice. Why do you think that industry does all the thing that it does to the "alternative," "pseudo," and all other "names" scientist that do not follow company line? Do you think that this is just so that you can be safe from bad doctors that will do you harm because they are all insane and snake oil salesmen's? Do you know that doctors themselves have a fear of losing their job for not following industry guidelines? Do you think "they" care about you? At the end of the day, the medicine did release us from infections with antibiotics and vaccines.

People are born with only two instinctive fears. One is the fear of falling, and other is of intense noises. Everything else you fear has been obtained during your lifetime and are usually generated by some circumstances and situations that have registered in your mind and emotions in a way that makes you feel scared. That is when our body responds with the 'fight or flight' response. Fear is the strongest emotion, and eventually it will condition our behavior. Fear is stronger than rational thinking because it is a conditioned evolutionary response for keeping us alive. For all animals and for our hominin ancestors some real fears where fear of becoming meal and fear from starvation. The humans might add the third one, and that was fear from the disease. Today we do not have to fear predation anymore and for most of the developed world fear of hunger does not exist. However, there is still fear from the disease. And where is fear there is manipulation? Some people are very good at utilizing the emotions of others for their own benefit. They like to call that marketing or propaganda or mainstream media. It is just emotional manipulation. In some cases, withholding the facts can have the same desired effect.

Don't get me wrong having profit in medicine is nothing bad. The problem arose when medicine became the part of larger hierarchical social structure system that is designed for widespread control and usage of people as a resource. Another part of the problem we face in medicine is philosophical in nature. The modern way of comprehension of reality is based on a belief system that human reason is superior force than nature. The other prevailing belief is that there is no such thing as life. Yes, you read that right. Scientific medicine does not believe that there is such thing in existence as life. Life is not life. There is no distinction between living and dead matter. The life is just dead matter arranged in such a manner to form the most complicated and structured machine in the universe that we perceive as life. It is just rearrangement of dead atoms. This belief system is in the essence of the theory of evolution and medicine and all of the science we have today. It is a basic principle that defines our entire civilization, not just medicinal practice. It is hard to explain so I will use an example. We can take a human organism and separate it into working parts. We will get brain, heart, lungs and so on. All of this organs are separated and do something for the organism. At the same time, we can take the average car and separate it into working parts too. We will get driving motor, wheels, hoods and so on. All of the parts are separated and do something for the car as a whole. So both the car and the man have many similar attributes. They have many functional parts. They can both move, they both need a constant supply of energy to work. When they do work they both heat up, and if they heat up too much, they need to stop and cool themselves. If they are left without energy, they both stop and eventually rust (get old) and die. Dying is actually not a real medical term. Because life does not exist and both cars and humans are just rearranged death mater they cannot die. They can just stop functioning.

Because our bodies are just stupid machines like any other car, we treat diseases, in the same manner, we treat broken cars. We have interventional treatments. This is belief system you will get in hospitals. This is actually great if you just had an accident and they need to save your life but terrible for anything else. This philosophy has a detrimental effect. Doctors actually do not treat diseases at all. They treat symptoms. For example, you have a cold, and your body raised the temperature to fight it. What will your MD prescribe? They will give you something to lower temperature and release you from pain. This will just make it more difficult for your immune system to fight, but now you do not have any symptoms. So are you healthy? If you do not have symptoms, you do not have the disease. You still have the virus, but you are feeling well, so you are fine. This is how modern medicine work. You might be full of toxins have high inflammation and who knows what but until you get some real problem like cancer or heart disease, guess what? You are healthy. Until they can detect any symptom, there is nothing they can do for you. They do not deal with promoting health and life. They are not health practicing industry. They deal with sickness. They deal with symptoms. Who deals with real diseases? Your body does. There are no cures in medicine just different pills. You can only help your body to heal and help it from becoming ill in the first place. The cures you get from doctors are not cures. They are treatments. When we combine these two beliefs that there is no such thing as life and that human reason is supreme force than nature we have something called allopathic (modern) medicine.

However, there is one crucial difference between machinery like automobiles and machinery like a human organism. Characteristic of a living organism is self-sufficiency. Living organisms, unlike machinery, can heal themselves and sustain themselves. They do not need a mechanic. If the car can self-repair and self-drive to the gasoline station, then the car would be a living creature. That is something modern allopathic medicine do not recognize. They treat every pain every symptom and every disease, but they do not treat the causes of the diseases and they do not treat the whole body holistically. Medicine is segregated to the specialist areas where every doctor is specialist in his domain and looks into his own organ where every problem gets its Latin name and list of medicine to prescribe. And that is it. Students learn this lists like they memorize lyrics from the songs and everyone sings his own song with a different prescription. That is as far as you will go in treatment in any hospital. The entire health fantasy is just propaganda for you so that you can feel safe and continue to give a big chunk of your income to the industry. They know that you don't care about your health as long as you are healthy and they wait for you to get some of the symptoms to feed on your anxiety. Modern medicine is like a parasite. It is just a business. It is too late for you when you get the first symptoms of chronic diseases. Remember this next sentence. There is no cure in pharmacy for anything. Your own body healing mechanism is the only cure. If you abuse it, don't expect purple magic pills. Only purple magic painkillers.

Around 100 years ago modern medicine was finally able to neutralize so-called empirical doctors or holistic or natural healers. They were called empirical because they have been utilizing only empirical observation without any form of science. Knowledge was carried down from one generation to another in the form of natural herbal and another form of folk medicine. In 1800s society was split between two forms of medicine and there was regulation of both forms with laws and restrictions equally. Patients had a choice of using both forms of treatment, the allopaths, and the empirics. The allopathic (modern) doctors called their approach heroic medicine and believed in the use of poisons to aggressively treat diseases. They called their practice scientific theory. They used three main techniques. They bled the body to drain out the bad toxins like in the Middle Age. In Middle Age plague treating practice was to cut open the veins leading to the heart. This in their mind would allow the disease to leave the body. The swellings associated with the Black Death also where cut open to allow the disease to leave. They continued to use this form of practice. Then they had been giving patients a huge doses of toxic heavy metals like mercury and lead to displace the original disease. They also used surgery which was the best method of them all. They scientifically studied human anatomy and believed in the same principle of aggressively treating diseases by cutting them out.

Empirical doctors believed in natural human body potential for self-healing and did not use any form of surgery. They did not even allow for piercing of the human skin in any form. So they never practiced surgery. In that time that was a brutal method without anesthetics and infection control. Even bad teeth were life-threatening and painful removal procedure without antibiotics. Allopaths did that surgery too. In that time most patients feared allopathic methods altogether and in not rare occasions patients did die from the cure. Empiric healers contrary to the doctors believed in stimulating the body's own defenses to heal itself instead. They used vegetable products, herbs, and nontoxic substances in small quantities. Usually, if treatment was not successful, they did not aggravate the state of disease, and if the patient did die, he died from the disease itself not from the "cure" like mercury or bleeding. The balance and coexistence of both medical branches remained equal to about the turn of the century when the new medical treatments emerged that were potentially very profitable. That possibility for huge profit is what changed everything in the upcoming years.

The American Medical Association was joined and influenced by strong financial and controlling forces and transformed medicine into the industry. An international banking cartel or in personal names Rockefeller, Morgan, Carnegie and Rothschild family financed surgery, radiation and synthetic drugs. Carnegie in later time sold out all of his businesses to Morgan and became a philanthropist. Rockefeller and Morgan were one of the founders and stockholders of Federal Reserve (a private bank that still controls the US and global economy by large extent) and were also heavy industry and oil industry monopolists. They were to become the business founders of the new emerging medical industry. A takeover of the medical schools allowed for a takeover of the entire medical industry. Carnegie, in particular, came into the picture and said that he would put finances. They invested tremendous amounts of money into the founding of the new industry, in particular into the schools that were complacent into cooperating with them. For the money, they spent they had a request to put some of their people into a board of directors to see that their money is spent wisely. It is not philanthropy when you give money so that you can put your agents in as executives. It is takeover that was represented as a philanthropy. What happened was that all of the major universities received large grants from these people and also accepted one or more of these people in the board of directors. Now, these people were not there to spread science and learning in pursuit of social well-being and human happiness. They were put there as a larger scheme of plans to ensure that the interest of the bankers are being fulfilled. Almost overnight schools where literally taken over. The schools did get large amounts of money, and they did spend it on new expensive equipment and build new buildings and new laboratories and hired more researchers and teachers. However, at the same time, they sold their interest to the growing industry called medicine dominated by newly founded pharmaceutical companies. Some of the money went directly into the pockets of Presidents of University's and other high ranking academia members as a bribe. If you are president of Harvard University for example, you are still open to "cooperation" especially if you need to develop the moral values that are in direct conflict with organized crime syndicates and banking cartels. You take the money and do as told. Physicians from that time onward in history would be taught pharmaceutical drugs and allopathic form of interventional medicine for the benefit of private financial interest of international banking cartel led by Rockefellers and Morgan.

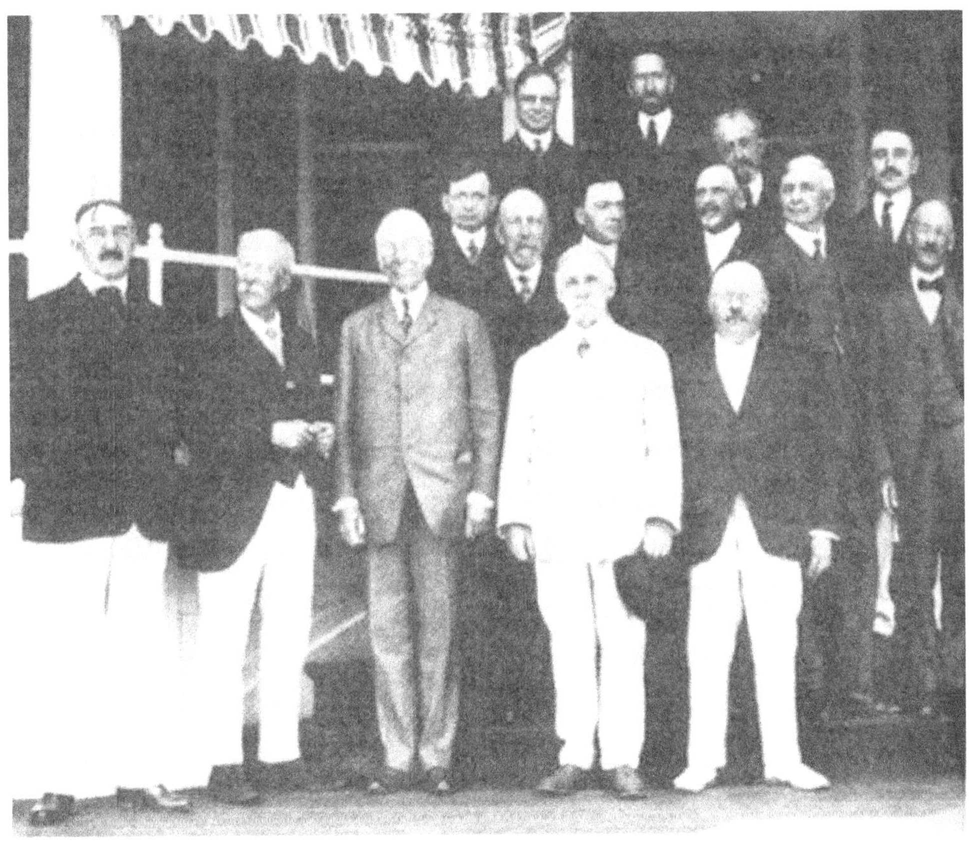

On the picture, you can see trustees of the General Educational Board, the first Rockefeller foundation at a retreat in Rockland, Maine, July in 1915. Beside

Rockefeller, in the middle, you can also see for instance Charles W. Eliot (former president of Harvard University), Harry Pratt Judson (President of University of Chicago) and many other "important" individuals that just by meeting in such arrangement have created something known as a conflict of interest.

It is amazing how little money really took to do it. By that time surgery became a more important aspect of allopathic medicine because of anesthesia and infection control and doctors advocated more and more the use and research into expensive operations as a cure for every disease where it can be implemented. Then the large and lucrative hospital system where constructed and radium fever swept medicine. Price of radium rose 1000% overnight. A drug industry grew from booming patented medicine. The schools changed education standards and licensing regulations to exclude the empirics. Only AMA approved doctors could legally practice medicine. The media campaign was launched to spread fear and associate empirics with quacks and danger. From that time and to this day schools of medicine represent an interest of banking cartel and not the interest of individuals. Average doctor in medical school get a great education, he knows a lot about drugs and surgery, but he does not know a one damn thing about nutrition. And he has learned to associate nutrition with quackery and to keep his mouth shut and to go with industry guidelines for fear of losing his six-figure salary. He has learned that the only thing that matter is what the big book from which he learns in school told him because that is science and everything else is evil. The average doctor is in the same mindset as someone that has been indoctrinated into the religious cult. He had a fear of death if he starts to think outside of the industry guidelines literally.

There is a high probability that he will lose his job for trying to help people. Then he is going to lose his house and then he is not going to be able to pay his student loan. Even if he knows what is going on eventually, he will accept the system and will defend it. He will give a Hippocratic oath, but he is not a natural doctor. Hippocrates himself was empirical healer with "passive" approach and believed that disease is caused by environmental factors, diet, and living habits. One of the "passive" quotes from oath "First do no harm" is: "I will use treatment to help the sick according to my ability and judgment, but never with a view to injury and wrong-doing. Neither will I administer a poison to anybody when asked to do so, nor will I suggest such a course. Similarly, I will not give to a woman fluorine to cause abortion. But I will keep pure and holy both my life and my art. I will not use the knife, not even, verily, on sufferers from stone, but I will give place to such as are craftsmen therein. Into whatsoever houses I enter, I will enter to help the sick, and I will abstain from all intentional wrong-doing and harm." Physicians of today do exactly everything in the opposite way and still use the oath. They will even consciously do you harm if that is what they were told to do. At the bare minimum, they will just be indifferent. Every drug on the market is poison and cannot be patented as a drug if it is not, or in other words if it has no side effects it cannot be registered and goes into over the counter supplement category.

Even to this day, the doctors are targeted for telling the truth. They learn in the college to keep their mouth shut. Dr. John McDougall story was a good example. He was almost thrown out of the medical school on couple occasions because he had hard time keeping his mouth shut. Then he was almost thrown out residency when he lost his cool after seeing one patient who had his third heart attack. He told the patient that he does not have a bright future if he does not shift to a starch-based diet of fruits and vegetables. His chief of Medicine called him in for a chat and told him that he embarrassed his attending doctor by talking about food and that he should never do that again if he needs to hold any job in the future. So he shut up for a while, and after he got his "ticket" the chief of Medicine for the residency University of Hawaii Dr. Schatz called him in again, and he said: "You know McDougall, I like you. I like your wife and your children. I think you have a great family, but I am afraid you are going to starve to death with your crazy ideas about vegetarian diet. You are not going to work anywhere, and the only patient you will ever collect are a bunch of bums and hippies." This is the same way that any form of organized crime function thru different forms of intimidation toward your family. McDougall told him he had a big fat abdomen but that he has to look himself in the mirror and that he will not treat chronic diseases with drugs and surgery. For people who do not know today open heart surgery cost is: $324,000. You just cannot make that kind of profit with the selling of sweet potatoes. McDougall problem was that he was raised in the poor American family where the highest principles were honesty, so he probably did not fit well in the medical industry. Fortunately, he was not that big to became a real target, so he lived full life. He later wrote the book named The Starch Solution.

I just use his situation for example of the functioning of the entire system. Industry targets systematically every conceivable threat with no exception. This was 1978, and to this day the situation is the same. McDougall even get kicked out of the Obesity Medicine Conference in San Francisco in 2016. He was asked to talk at the conference but the medical conference people required for all the speakers to submit the slides and videos for approval. Initially they thought that his approach was based on the Mediterranean diet but when they realized that it is not Mediterranean diet they thought that it was, the full meat, alcohol and cheese false Mediterranean diet and that instead, it was really poor people low-fat vegan starch-based diet they uninvited him with excuse that he is not willing to be "politically correct". He also got a law passed in 2011. He testified before

Senate committee on the need to educate medical students on human nutrition. The bill was SB 380 Continuing medical education. It was passed in California Congress, and it was signed by Governor so it became the law in California to force the 11 medical schools to teach nutrition to medical students. However, the medical industry does not have an interest in healing the people, so the implementation of the law was given to the Medical Board in California. They fulfill the law by putting one paragraph in their newsletter once a year about nutrition.

This battle for human lives are real, but it is waged behind the scenes. What most people are familiar is just propaganda. Doctors are good, they have to pledge a Hippocratic oath, there are there to heal you and help you, and of course one day the medicine is going to deliver us from all diseases. In reality, it is completely opposite and sometimes completely in your face that it is pathetic. We can just remember the examples like "McGovern Report." In 1977 the "McGovern Report" came out. George McGovern was former Democratic Senator from South Dakota who in 1972 suffered a presidential defeat to Richard Nixon, but he also was in the head of the committee that released the first Dietary Guidelines in the US. Before that, it was as it is now. Meat and sugar. At 1977 everything you read in this book was known. Every single thing. Evan before that. What was so evil about the report. It basically stated that we should eat more whole grains, more fruits, more vegetables, less meat, less dairy, at least less whole fat dairy, sugar and so on. It did not advocate a vegan diet, but it was basically the step in a similar direction. These new guidelines on eating were expected to have similar health-changing effects as the 1964 Surgeon General's Report on Smoking. The McGovern Report found and this is a quote from a report itself that: "There is a great deal of evidence, and it continues to accumulate, which strongly implicates and, in some instances, proves that the major causes of death and disability in the United States are related to the diet we eat. I (Dr. Hegsted of Harvard School of Public Health) include coronary artery disease, which accounts for nearly half the deaths in the United States, several of the most important forms of cancer, hypertension, diabetes, and obesity as well as other chronic diseases." Industry and a big chunk of senators called report big conspiracy theory and that McGovern Committee believes in depriving people of what they like. This was from an official record of the committee hearing, and later the same story was pushed in mainstream media. If you don't believe conspiracy theories and watch mainstream media here is one example of the mindset of industry people. At that time The Salt institute warned that: "If people eat healthier, we would have more old people to take care of"..., "simultaneously increasing the cost of care of old people which comes under the category of healthcare expenditures."

Rulers of people don't like old ones because they do not produce and just suck off the resources that rulers want for themselves. It is better for them and for the economy when people die at 60 just before pension, and it is even better when they spend their entire savings on heart surgery and chemotherapy before they die. It would not be cost effective for rulers to have masses of people regularly living to 90. This planet in their mindset is already overpopulated. The other industries also went ballistic especially meat and egg. They warn that: "If Dietary Goals are mowed forward and promoted as a present norm the entire sectors of the food industry –meat, dairy, sugar, and others may be so severely damaged that when it is realized that Dietary Goals are ill-advised, as surely will be the discovery, production recovery may be out of reach." However, the food industry did not stop this report. This report was eventually stopped at the highest political level. The level that sees people as a resource.

The companies that made up pharmaceutical industry are one of the largest corporations in the world, and by a great extent are owned by the same people that own the big international banks and other large industries. They are not a separate entity. They are one level of multiple levels of the larger industry owned by a small number of individuals. The tale of Big Pharma is the exact same as the story of Big Government, Big Oil, Big Agri-Chem Giants, Big Heavy Industry, Big Military Industrial Complex. The governing stockholders of all those main industries are exactly the same people. Big Money coming from the global central banking cartel owns and operates all the Fortune 500 companies.

The Rockefeller family privatized the medical industry in the United States back in the beginning of the 20th century. From that time onward, it never stopped spreading through the entire world. The real history of the last couple of centuries is that there is central monopolistic ruling elite made out of handful of these oligarch families, primarily from Europe and the United States, that have been influencing governments and instigating wars to ruthlessly consolidate and maximize both power and control over the resources (especially oil) and entire global population. Big pharma is just one part of it. Big Pharma's top eleven companies made net profits in just one decade from 2003 to 2012 of nearly three-quarters of a trillion dollars, and that's net profit alone not sales. The most of those biggest pharmaceuticals are headquartered in the US – including the top four, Johnson & Johnson (#39 on Fortune 500 list), Pfizer (#51), Merck (#65) and Eli Lilly (#129) along with Abbott (#152) and Bristol Myers Squibb (#176). In 2014, total pharmaceutical revenues worldwide had exceeded one trillion US dollars for the first time. Because Big Pharma sometimes outright owns and largely controls today's most prominent medical journals, and mainstream media is owned by the same people too, spreading false propaganda, disinformation and lies is common practice. Similar to shady personnel moving shamelessly in and out of governmental public service to think tanks to universities to private law to corporations to lobbyists, the same applies to heads of the FDA moving to and from Big Pharma.

Unfortunately, the government has been taken over by special interest groups and not today but more than 100 years ago. First Rockefeller, Morgan and Carnegie gained control of the teaching system. Then they gave AMA power to exclude all of the empirics and doctors they do not like from practicing. Then took over entire drug testing process by heavily influencing medical publications that review those drugs. They also gained control of the media. Finally, they extended their control over FDA that supposed to verify those drugs safety and efficacy. Actually, it started more than 100 years ago. Standard Oil Co. Inc. was an established in 1870 by John D. Rockefeller. At that time, it was the biggest oil refinery in the world. Rockefeller was also a psychopath, a supporter of capitalism that loved social Darwinism or used it as a justification. He was often quoted as saying: "The growth of a large business is merely the survival of the fittest." Soon after the discovery of oil in Titusville, Pennsylvania, the 24-year-old Rockefeller joined the oil business. First in 1863 by investing in a Cleveland refinery. In 1870, he created the Standard Oil Company of Ohio with his younger brother William, Henry Flagler and some additional investors. He made a secret agreement with railroad monopolist that allowed Standard Oil to produce a large amount of oil to achieve economies of scale. With a never-ending supply of money from Bank of Cleveland (Rothschild owned bank) and secured railroad deals he rapidly managed to intimidate all the rivals to buy them out. Standard Oil finally dominated 90 percent of the market of the US. Ten year later he moved the central Standard Oil's headquarters to New York City where they have their own political lobbyist and governors in place. Because of this monopoly that were spreading from banks to oil to everywhere, the U.S. Supreme Court ruled that Standard Oil in 1911 get dismantled because it violated federal anti-trust laws. The company was dismantled into 34 separate companies. However, Rockefeller was still the owner of them all. This in reality, did nothing. Some of these companies later became Chevron, Amoco, Conoco, ExxonMobil. What happened was that dismantling them made more money because combining individual worth of them all actually worth more than Standard Oil. Some of them tripled in value in early years making Rockefeller the first publicly recognized billionaire with a fortune that was equal to 2 percent of entire U.S. economy. In time company diversified, even more, became like octopus but the owner was still Rockefeller. We might have Fortune 500, and it might look that there are many companies on the free market, but the owners are still the same just this time in secret. And today it is on the global level. We are going to analyze here just petrochemical business that connects Rockefeller with medicine.

His own father William Avery Rockefeller was a snake oil salesman. He even posed as a deaf and mute peddler with miracle herbal remedies. He was dubbed as "Devil Bill." He also posed as an eye and ear specialist Dr. William Levingston. In 1885 he even secretly married another woman beside the first one that fathered John. John never publicly acknowledged his father bigamist life. In fact, if we look with little more detail in his biography, we will see that he was notorious horse stealer and conman of every kind, which spend most of his money in bordellos. Because of a number of indictments, he constantly was moving from town to town. He also raped a hired girl in 1849 for which he was indicted. Most of money he made by selling his miraculous cancer cure and another product named "Wonder Working Liniment" which he sold at two dollars for the bottle as a laxative. It consisted of crude petroleum from which lither oils had been removed so what was left was a heavy solution of lube oil, tar, and paraffin. He passed away at the age of 95 in Freeport, Illinois. However, he also was never buried there. He was buried in an unmarked grave as Dr. William Levingston. This "Dr." had made it possible for "Devil Bill" to sell his elixir for many diseases. In that period there were many diseases especially because of bad hygiene and alcohol abuse. So what was his miraculous cancer cure of magic?

It was just stone oil known as petroleum. It was found in salt wells at Tarentum near Pittsburgh. Owner of the land named Samuel Kier at first simply dumped the useless oil into the nearby Pennsylvania Main Line Canal, but after an oil slick caught fire, he saw a way to profit from this otherwise worthless byproduct. He started to collect the oil in bottles and have been selling it as a patent medicine charging $0.50 per bottle. He named it "Rock Oil" and later "Seneca Oil." Seneca was an Indian tribe. One of the first wholesale traders who started to buy this oil from him was "Devil Bill," William Avery Rockefeller. Kier later established America's first oil refinery in Pittsburgh. Nevertheless, the best marketing of this oil was done by Dr. William Levingston, the "famous expert in the field of tumors." He was pushing the product as a cure for all tumors if the disease was still in the early stages and have not progressed too far. The same sentence you will hear today in modern oncology. "Devil Bill" was able to sell one bottle of the stuff for 25$, and in that time that was the two-month salary of the average worker.

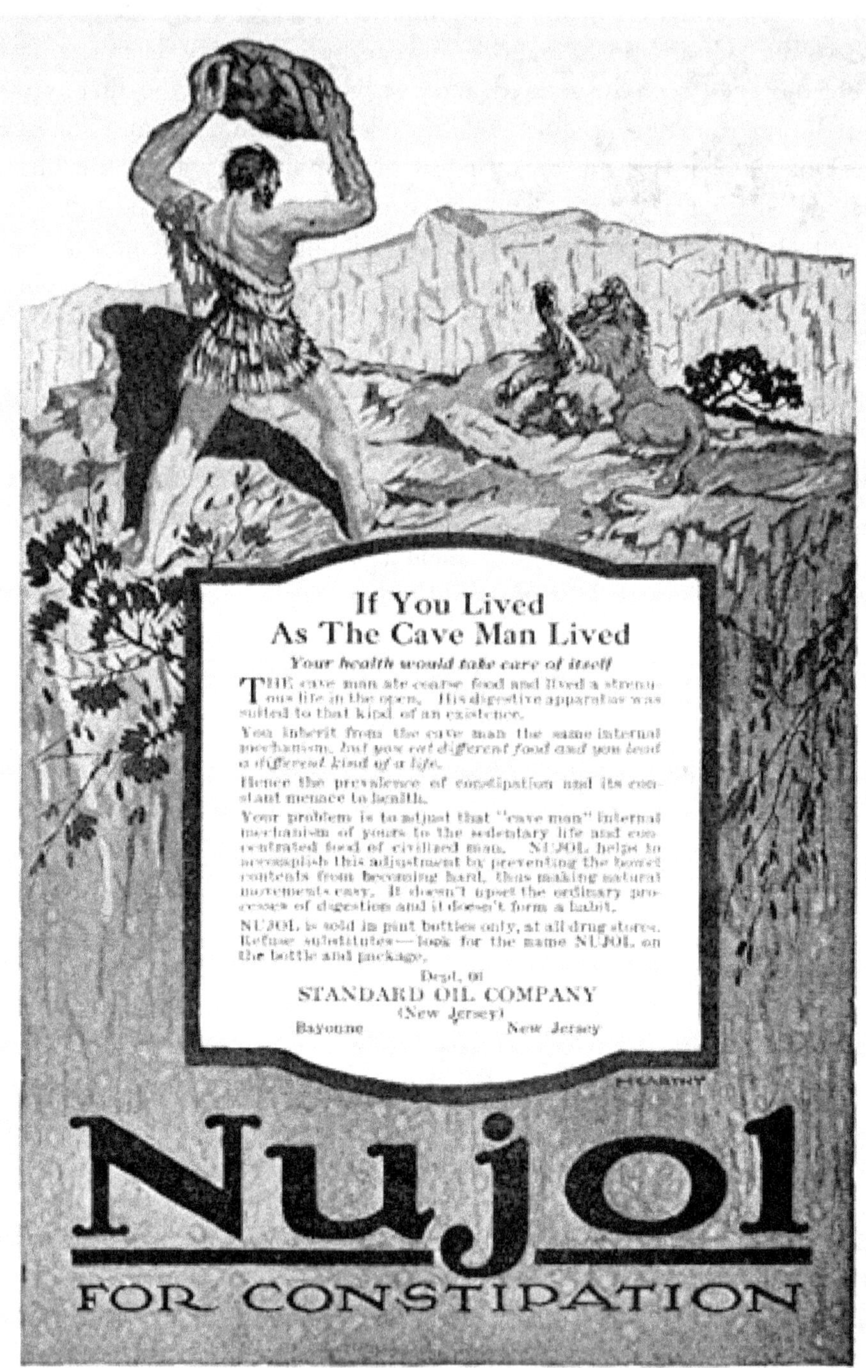

Send for booklet, "THE RATIONAL TREATMENT OF CONSTIPATION." Write your name and address plainly on the margin below.

His son John continued father business. Standard Oil had begun to manufacture one more "miraculous" cure from oil, which was in sales until recently. It was the type of oil that was used as a laxative. As same as before it was made of crude petroleum from which lither oils had been removed so what was left was a heavy solution of lube oil, tar, and paraffin. In Standard Oil, they packed this in small bottles and named it "Nujol."

It was manufactured by Stanco Incorporated in Jersey as part of Standard Oil. The second chemical Stanco was producing was insecticide FLIT. Even in the beginning, there were no differences between the oil industry and the chemical industry and the medical industry. It was the same company under the different names. No Fortune 500. Only Fortune 1. In reality, it did not matter to the "Devil Bill" or his son John that the oil that they are selling is actually a poison as long as they made money out of it. In the same factory, they had been manufacturing both insecticide poison FLIT and oil sludge cure elixir Nujol for human consumption. Nujol was very dangerous because it was leeching the minerals out of the body. It was well known fact that mineral oils create mucus that outlines the intestines preventing the absorption of water. Just as mineral oil limits the absorption of water through the intestines, it can also interfere with the absorption of other nutrients especially minerals and also medicines and vitamins. Mineral oil may cause diarrhea, leading to dehydration and nutrient loss and it was especially that property that was utilized as a laxative. Potassium and salt loss from diarrhea can cause potentially harmful conditions, including abnormal heart rhythms and muscle cramps but that was not important to John he just wanted to make money, and he did. From one barrel of oil which had priced at that time of 2$, Stanco Incorporated was able after the boiling to fill around 1000 one ounce bottles of this sludge. Big wholesale distributors of medicinal products had been buying this for the price of 21 cents per bottle. Standard Oil manufacturing cost was one-fifth of the one cent. This line of business might be ridiculous for the company that by that time had already expanded into the overseas markets, particularly Western Europe and Asia, and after a while it was selling even more oil abroad than in the US. Rockefeller, in addition to his role as the head of Standard Oil, also invested in numerous companies in manufacturing, transportation and other industries and owned major iron mines and extensive tracts of timberland.

What was the next Rockefeller push into the chemical and drug industry was the creation of a trust for entire wholesale drug market between 1939 and 1949 in control of Rockefellers. After the success of Nujol and tested and proven fact that you can sell anything with good propaganda and with plans to put the entire currently rising patented drug chemical industry into the control, the next step was to incorporate all of the medical schools and governmental institutions into the line of the industry. They applied for a federal charter for the Rockefeller Foundation in the US Senate in 1910, for pushing their philanthropic endeavors for which they separated the flat amount of 100 million dollars. When American president at that time William Howard Taft, seen the amount for the spending of the endowment for philanthropy he realized that it has nothing to do with the philanthropy. He even had been secretly meeting with Rockefeller lobbyist (three inaugural trustees, Junior, Gates and Harold Fowler McCormick). Because Taft and some of the ministers in his government recognized the secret agenda, they pushed hard against the endowment. They then, Senior and Gates, withdrew the bill from Congress in order to pass it as state charter. They managed to do this with the support of Rothschild agent from Germany named Robert Ferdinand Wagner I. He was a Democratic U.S. Senator from New York from 1927 to 1949. Born in Prussia, Wagner migrated with his family to the United States in 1885 and later became senator of the state of New York by Rockefeller money. Wagner was later a leader of the New Deal Coalition and strong supporter of President Franklin D. Roosevelt. In 1913, New York Governor William Sulzer approved a state charter for the foundation with Junior becoming the first president and ranking Rockefeller "the greatest philanthropist in American history". I won't go into more detail because it will take an entire book to do good historical analysis of the way the elite structures of a control function, but one more thing we need to pay the attention is something called Eugenics.

Eugenics (from Greek εὐγενής eugenics 'well-born' from εὖ eu, 'good, well' and γένος genos, 'race, stock, kin'). It is a form of philosophy if you like that aims at improving the genetic quality of a human population. It began with Plato suggesting applying the same principles of selective breeding that give rise to an increased yield of crops after the Neolithic Revolution to humans themselves around 400 BC. He wanted to create guardian race. The big chunk of culture in Ancient Greece was similar with glorifying human body and perfection and in some places like Sparta practices like throwing deformed and week babies into the pits was common practice. When a cousin of Darwin Sir Francis Galton started to promote those theories with increased vigor, elite oligarch loved it. Galton further insisted that if genetically healthy and talented individuals only marry other more superior individuals, the end outcome would be considered more fit and talented offspring. It is the same logic that was practiced in agriculture for thousands of years giving us all of our modern foods. However, the elite loved it. This bizarre theory was in some sense logical and applicable to humans as well as to other animals. For example, all of the different dog breeds are just product of selective breeding. Eventually, it transformed to well-accepted philosophy of eugenics.

The philosophy that resulted in pushing for feminism, abortion, forced sterilizations, euthanasia and in some cases even full-blown infanticide. It is the same philosophy that exists today. For example, when a country of Iceland brags about the healing of Down syndrome that is just eugenics in practice. This was all in early years even before World War 2 and had nothing to do with the Nazi party and their philosophy of racism. Actually, Hitler himself look at academia in the US as a model for population control and dealing with "unfits." Before World War 2 this philosophy was so accepted as a part of social Darwinism in most of the elite circles and academia that it got massive funding from hereditary elite families such as Carnegie and Rockefellers. Who do you think gave funds for the coordination and implementation of the program in which Josef Mengele personally worked before his infamous experiments at Auschwitz? Go and learn some of the history if you do not know the answer. From 1930 the Rockefeller Foundation contributed substantial financial support to the Kaiser Wilhelm Institute of Anthropology, Human Heredity, and Eugenics. That was the institute that later conducted eugenics experiments in the Third Reich. The modern eugenics was not something Nazi party accepted as a racist ideology. It was philosophy first practiced in ancient Greece, and in modern time it emerged in the UK at the beginning of the 20th century and then spread to the US and other countries like Canada and most of Western Europe. Ordinary people were not interested in this, but academia and elite was and still is. When you see someone talking about the overpopulation of the planet he is emerged into this philosophy. It is still alive especially in ruling elite and political spectrum. Today they are using subtler measures instead of sterilization like abortion pills, but back in the day, they have actually advocated measures as forced sterilization. The Rockefeller Foundation provided funds to Nazi racial studies even after it was obvious that the research mentioned above had been used to rationalize the demonizing of Jews and other groups. All away up to 1939 the Rockefeller Foundation was funding research used to support Nazi racial science studies at the Kaiser Wilhelm Institute of Anthropology, Human Heredity, and Eugenics (KWIA). Reports submitted to Rockefeller did not hide what these studies were being used to justify, but Rockefeller continued the funding and refrained from criticizing this research so closely derived from Nazi ideology. This movement never died. It is the philosophical driving force for an entire elite structure from a time of Plato.

In the 1950s, the Rockefellers restructured eugenics movement in their own family offices in America. They had just used different more delicate names for it like abortion, woman rights and population-control. Because of all of the bad association that word eugenics now had after the WW2 and Nazi eugenic experiments they decided to spin the name to Society for the Study of Social Biology. This is the current organization name. The spin-off. Ok, social biology meaning social Darwinism meaning racism and not just racism but selective breeding and sterilization and population reduction and control. The Rockefeller Foundation also had provided funds to eugenics movement in Britain. In the 1960s, the Eugenics Society of England chose something they called crypto-eugenics. Crypto meaning is hidden. What they stated in their reports is that they will no longer use the word but will continue the program by stealth. They are going to use social justice and other non-governmental agencies to push for population reduction and other measures believed by philosophy.

By assistance from the Rockefellers, the Eugenics Society of England created an organization that still exist and do their job today named International Planned Parenthood Federation, which for 12 years had no other address than the Eugenics Society. Within the Bureau of Social Hygiene, and just the name Social Hygiene gives me the creeps, that is another Rockefeller eugenics foundation. John D. Rockefeller also anonymously financed the infamous eugenicist, racist and abortion lobbyist Margaret Sanger's American Birth Control League, Birth Control Clinical Research Bureau, and already mention Planned Parenthood of America. Sanger was also "mother" of modern feminism with the belief that empowering the woman will lower the birth rate and was "mother" of an idea of legalized abortion. Rockefellers later founded the whole endeavor. And why would the Rockefellers finance feminism? Well, they required females to work so that they could tax half of the population more and that will also lower the average income meaning more work from everyone for less money meaning more to the elite. Their children would now be without supervision and will have to go into state-run schools. They could then be taught whatever is necessary to be loyal to the state. However, the main reason is that the nuclear family would take a nose dive and the birth rate with it. Sanger was also the initiator of The Negro Project. It was a social control mechanism designed to depopulate negroids. In a 1939 message to Clarence Gamble, she wrote: "We do not want word to go out that we want to exterminate the Negro population and the minister is the man who can straighten out that idea if it ever occurs to their more rebellious members." In 1939, Sanger changed the name of her Clinical Research Bureau to the Birth Control Clinical Research Bureau, both integral institutions to the Negro Project, which became the Planned Parenthood Federation of America in 1942. The same foundation that today provide the woman with birth control pills for free. Rockefeller family that has as much control as it does, plus all other elites and their obsession with eugenics is a great concern for a common man.

Their obsession with this philosophy have escalated to the global scale. Considering Rockefellers and Rothschilds connection with the creation of to the United Nations and their role in its creation. Population control and reduction are one of the main concerns of the UN. Imagine that. They fund a variety of different organizations under the UN umbrella to be stealthy. They adopted the England stealth model now. For example, the United Nations Population Fund. Sven Burmester, a representative of the U.N. organization, stated his support for the practices of China's population control programs publicly. He said: "China has had the most successful family planning policy in the history of mankind in terms of quantity, and with that, China has done mankind a favor." The Rockefellers themselves are only agents or partners of individuals at even higher places. It is the entire elite that supports this philosophy.

The point of this analysis is that we understand logically that the same people behind eugenics are the same people behind industry or let say shareholders of Big Pharma that supposedly wants to heal people from disease. The same people who see common people like cattle for selective breeding. Transhumanism, for example, is a modern form of belief that is associated with eugenics. Most transhumanists have the same views nevertheless distance themselves from the term "eugenics" (preferring "germinal choice" or "reprogenetics"). It is the same system that pushes for depopulation of the planet on different fronts with different measures including war. Even fetal screening can be viewed as a form of modern eugenics because it may lead to the abortion of a child with undesirable traits. In Iceland, with prenatal screening, they managed to "heal" Down syndrome. The way Eugenics and Social Darwinism work is that there is no mercy or good or wrong or evil. The strong shall inherit the Earth not the meek. Christian philosophy of altruism like Matthew 5:5: "Blessed are the meek: for they shall inherit the earth", is in their mind just childish. Who weeps for the Neanderthal? The way slave owners looked at racism was just in the line of the fact that there was no military in Africa or nothing else to pose any real difficulty for enslavement. In Ancient Rome and Ancient Greece all of the slaves were white. Talking about feelings and morals is absolute in Social Darwinism and it has nothing to do with the color of the skin or nationality or religion. It is more complex and more scientific philosophy then just racism, but racism can be in some sense a part of it.

The only real question here was the Rockefeller fully independent as a capitalist individual or did he became an agent of larger banking cartel from Europe? I think that the answer is mix of both, but that is just my opinion based on some of the economic arrangements that he had with the National City Bank of Cleveland. Rockefeller as a successful man that did everything in the line of Social Darwinism without any regrets obsessed by greed obscures the fact that from the day one the Rockefellers began advancing towards a complete oil monopoly in the United States with almost the unlimited funding that came from the National City Bank of Cleveland. The question is how much of the

Rockefeller wealth may be attributed to old John ruthlessness because the National City Bank of Cleveland, was recognized in Congressional reports as one of the three Rothschild banks in the US. Rockefeller had support and the supervision of Jacob Schiff of Kuhn, Loeb & Company who had been born in the Rothschild house in Frankfort. He was Rothschild main representative in the US. With the seed money of unlimited amounts from the National City Bank of Cleveland, John D. Rockefeller soon laid claim to the title of the most ruthless American, but with full unlimited funding from old ruling monopolist from Europe. Rothschild family had backed him but to which extent I could not tell. Was he just an agent or he was in some form a partner in crime at the end is not relevant to us. This kind of deals are secret to full extent.

The world financial structure, on the other hand, cannot be hidden organization, like other policies. First on the list are the major Swiss Banks. These are not ordinary banks but survivors of the old Venetian-Genoese banking elite. Then there is the British combine with a center in the Bank of England. From a Bank of England, it operates to control merchant banks through Rothschild's and the Oppenheimer's and to hold full power over their Canadian territory through the Royal Bank of Canada and the Bank of Montreal. The Bank of England establishes colonial banking constructions in the United States through the Federal Reserve System (privately owned bank). The Boston Brahmin families who made their wealth in the opium trade, the Delanos, Kissinger network headquartered in the Rockefeller Bank, American Express, Chase Manhattan Bank all represent a form of the old Rothschild representatives in the United States, which also includes Kuhn, Loeb Company and Lehman Brothers. Then there is also the world great five of grain trade that controls food distribution.

The part of Rockefeller monopoly on chemical and medicine industries came into fulfillment after the WW2. And this happened on the global scale, not just US. Rockefeller and Rothschild cooperation made this into reality. On the other side of Atlantic, the international drug and chemical cartel, I.G. Farben, called "a state within a state" was created in 1925 as Interessen Gemeinschaft Farbenindustrie Aktien Gesellschaft, usually known as I.G. Farben, which simply meant "The Cartel." IG Farben had an absolute monopoly in manufacturing all of the chemical products all the way to the WW2. They were one if not the crucial financiers of rearmament of Germany with a special interest in oil production for German new mechanized army. It had at first started in 1904. Six main chemical companies in Germany made agreement to form the one final cartel, merging Badische Anilin, Bayer, Agfa, Hoechst, Weiler-ter-Meer, and Griesheim-Electron. The main financing came from the Rothschild family, who remained represented by their German banker, Max Warburg, of M.M. Warburg Company, Hamburg. He later directed the German Secret Service through World War I and was a private economic consultant to the Kaiser. Meanwhile, the Kaiser was overthrown after losing the war but Max Warburg was not exiled with him. He was above the politics as an agent of a higher power, so he never went to Holland. He instead became the economic consultant to the new government. He also represented Germany at the Paris Peace Conference. Max Warburg spent relaxing times rebuilding family ties with his brother, Paul Warburg, who, after conscripting the Federal Reserve Act at Jekyll Island, were controlling the US banking system through the war. He was also present in Paris as Woodrow Wilson's financial advisor. Two brothers were controlling two different banking systems in countries that supposedly are at war with one another. Before World War 2, Max Warburg served on the board of directors of I.G. Farben. His brother Paul Warburg served on the board of directors of I.G. Farben's specifically owned by American subsidiary. Warburg family was a prominent German and American banking family of German Jewish and originally Venetian Jewish descent at which point they bore the surname Del-Banco. However, at one time, the Warburg bank in Hamburg was about to collapse in 1857. The Rothschild family injected vast amounts of money into it becoming the new owners of the bank. From this period forward M.M. Warburg Bank and its partners operated effectively as Rothschild family fronts. The first member actually who was known to use the name "Rothschild" was Izaak Elchanan Rothschild, born in 1577. The name Rothschild in Yiddish means Red Coat. I.G. Farben quickly became a company that had the net worth of six billion marks, controlling more than five hundred firms.

When the Weimar Republic began to collapse, I.G. officials, seeing the writing on the wall, started a close cooperation with Adolf Hitler, providing enormous amounts of required funds and political influence. The progress of the I.G. Farben cartel had incited the interest and spread to other industrialists as well. Henry Ford was fairly impressed and set up a German branch of Ford Motor Company. I.G. Farben purchased forty percent of the stock. I.G. Farben next built an American subsidiary, called American I.G., in cooperation with Standard Oil of New Jersey. In 1930, Standard Oil declared that it had acquired a liquor monopoly in Germany, a deal that they had with I.G. Farben. It was already spreading into Europe food industry. After the Nazi party came to power, John D. Rockefeller hired his own press agent Ivy Lee to Hitler, to work as a full-time consultant on the rearmament of Germany. They had already decided to rearm Germany and to have WW2 so even back then necessary steps for setting up World War 2 had begun. Standard Oil next constructed large refineries in Germany for the Nazis and continued to supply them with oil during World War 2. In 1939 Frank Howard, a vice-president of Standard Oil visited Germany and made some arrangements. He later testified: "We did our best to work out complete plans for a modus vivendi which would operate throughout the term of the war, whether we came in or not. "

Although his name is hardly known, Frank Atherton Howard was in that time one of the main agents that directed Standard Oil operations. He also was director of the research committee at Sloan Kettering Institute during the 1930s. He was Rockefellers agent and was good at his job. His appointee at Sloan Kettering, Dusty Rhoads, managed the research that created chemotherapy. During the WW2, Rhoads headed the Chemical Warfare Service in Washington at U.S. Army Headquarters. The same men researched a cure for cancer and chemicals for the killing of people in wars, sound familiar by now. Men who also works for Rockefeller syndicate. It was Frank Howard that influenced both Alfred Sloan and Charles Kettering of General Motors in 1939 to give large donations to the Cancer Center, which then took on their names. Frank Howard second wife was a leading member of the British aristocracy, the Duchess of Leeds. I am writing his marital status just so that we can understand what government, aristocracy, democracy, capitalism and so on in reality is. It is all the same. Frank Howard was the key executive in managing relationships among Standard Oil and I.G. Farben working to coordinate the interest of both companies. He led in the research in the advancement of artificial rubber, which was vital to Germany in the Second World War. He later even wrote a book, "Buna Rubber." And IG Farben was also direct supporter without any secrecy of Nazi Party.

At a conference of German industrialists with Nazis like Hermann Goering and Heinrich Himmler, held on the 20 February 1933, IGF contributed 400,000 reichsmarks to the Nazi Party. It was the largest single amount of the total sum of 3 million reichsmarks raised at this meeting by German industrialists for the Nazi Party's election campaign. I.G. Farben contributed four and a half million reichsmarks to the Nazi Party in 1933. By 1945, I.G. had provided the Nazi Party with 40 million reichsmarks, a sum which matched all donations by I.G. to all other beneficiaries during that period. Now let me ask this question. Do you think that American or English governments did not know what is going on and from where the money are coming from? They planned and financed the entire WW2 by design. For example, without the clear help of Standard Oil, the Nazi air force would never be able to fly in the first place. The planes that made up the Luftwaffe needed tetraethyl lead gasoline in order to be able to fly. At the time, only General Motors, Standard Oil and Du Pont, had the ability to produce this vital substance. All companies outside of Germany. In 1938, Walter C. Teagle, the director of Standard Oil, accommodated Hermann Schmitz of I.G. Farben to obtain 500 tons of tetraethyl lead from Ethyl, a British Standard Oil subsidiary. One year later, Schmitz returned to London and purchased an extra

15 million dollars worth of value of tetraethyl lead. Then back in Germany that was turned into aviation gasoline for Luftwaffe.

It was in 1927 when Standard Oil and IG Farben founded the company Standard IG Farben. Standard passed to IG Farben the patents about the coal hydrogenation processes and the Germans gave them the patents how to manufacture synthetic rubber. While the European powers wanted to avoid the growth of German industry after WW1, the US companies spent huge sums of money to rebuild Germany and U.S. government never ratified the Versailles Treaty. Actually, not the government of US but the deep state power behind. They even sold German bonds in the US financial market. The whole episode was so blatant that it was almost unbelievable. One of the most important players in this "business" was the Union Banking Corporation of George H. Walker. He named his son-in-law, Prescott Bush, grandfather of US president George W. Bush, director of the firm. His grandson American President at the time George W. Bush was in the update 3.0 holding hands with Israeli Prime Minister and talking about the unity of American and Israeli people in „war of terror" forgetting the fact that his grandpa Prescott was using Jewish slave labor in his steel labor manufacturing plant at the Auschwitz. In update 1.0 Prescott father Samuel P. Bush longtime president of Buckeye Steel Castings company that was owned by Frank Rockefeller, the brother of John D. Rockefeller supplied parts for Edward Henry Harriman railroads which in return provided rail shipments for John's Standard Oil who in return got monopoly by financing from the Rothschild banks. Samuel son Prescott as the managing director of a Nazi steel manufacturing plant in Poland called Celestion Consolidated Steel who in update 2.0 forward American financing to his German partner Fritz Thyssen trough Union Banking Corporation in New York. Fritz Thyssen arranged a contract with IG Farben for free Jewish slave labor in Bush steel labor manufacturing plant at the Auschwitz concentration camp. In update 2 Prescott Busch and Averell Harriman (son of railroad baron E. H. Harriman, 48th Governor of New York and a core member of the group of foreign policy elders known as "The Wise Men" and Skull and Bones member) get caught under the trading with the enemy act as the US government moved in and seized all of the shares in Union Banking Corporation. In update 4.0 Prescott son first George Bush is director of the CIA. George pushed drug king Manuel Noriega on the CIA payroll and allowed tons of cocaine to hit the streets of America via the Panama Canal. In update 5.0 George son the second George Bush becomes partners with Osama bin Laden older brother Salem bin Laden in a Texas oil company called Arbusto energy. Also in update 5, we have an introduction to the George shady younger brother Neil Bush ripping off the elderly in the Silverado Saving and Loan scandal that cost US taxpayers 1.3 billion dollars. In the final update 6.0, we have George W. Bush, American President, visiting a death camp of Auschwitz to give a speech of "resisting the power of evil" where his grandfather helped build the Bush Family fortune on free Jewish slave labor. George Herbert Walker maternal grandfather of President George H. W. also got large contracts with the Germans, before and after 1933. In the board of his Walkers American Shipping and Commerce Company with its Hamburg-America Line was Emil Helfferich, member of Freundeskreis Reichsführer- SS and until end of WW2 President of Deutsch-Amerikanische Petroleum Gesellschaft, later ESSO, and Vacuum Oil Company in Hamburg.

The main problem for Germany's attack on the Soviet Union was the need for fuel for tanks and airplanes. Thanks to the patents of Standard Oil, the Germans could produce fuel from their own coal, but this was not enough. After the battle started in Europe, the English became annoyed about US shipments of vital materials to Nazi Germany. Standard Oil instantly transferred the registration of their entire fleet to Panama to avoid British search or seizure. These ships moved to bring oil to Tenerife, where they refueled German tankers for shipment to Hamburg. This deception was exposed on March 31, 1941, when the U.S. State Department issued a full report on refueling terminals in Mexico and Central and South America. What happened then? Nothing happened. There is no report of any form of action being taken because this all was planned on a higher level than just U.S. government.

A brief side note, however, is that on April 17, 1945 the Chase National Bank was put on trial in federal court on charges of having broken the Trading with the Enemy Act by changing German marks into US dollars. Because multiple nations rejected German currency throughout the war, the Nazis used international banks like Rockefellers Chase National to exchange the currency into money that would be accepted like dollars, and this would then have allowed them to purchase much need materials to further prolong the war. In the sense of the blunt opinions from Adolf Hitler himself on Jewish control in Germany, it would be challenging to explain the role of I.G. Farben in the Nazi era. Why? Because I.G. Farben was mostly controlled by Jewish bankers meaning Rothschilds in particular. During the 1920s it was accused by Nazis of being an "international capitalist Jewish company." Peter Hayes comprehensive study of I.G. Farben points that in 1933 it had ten Jews on its governing boards and do not forget, it was formed by Rothschild financing. The same company that had bought the patent for the pesticide Zyklon B, in the 1920s and later distributed it to the gas chambers of Auschwitz. Beside a synthetic oil and rubber plant at Auschwitz, the company also conducted drug experiments on live inmates. This apparatus utilized as much electricity as the entire city of Berlin, and more than 25,000 camp inmates died during its construction. I.G. Farben ultimately constructed its own concentration camp, known as Monowitz, which was closer to the factory in order to reduce the need to move already starving and on the brink of death prisoners several miles lowering the efficiency of their work. The same company that gives us aspirin. On a picture you can see the concentration camp constructed for the I.G. Farben Monowitz and bellow the camp the headquarters of the I.G. Farben intact by war and the American bombs and not by accident.

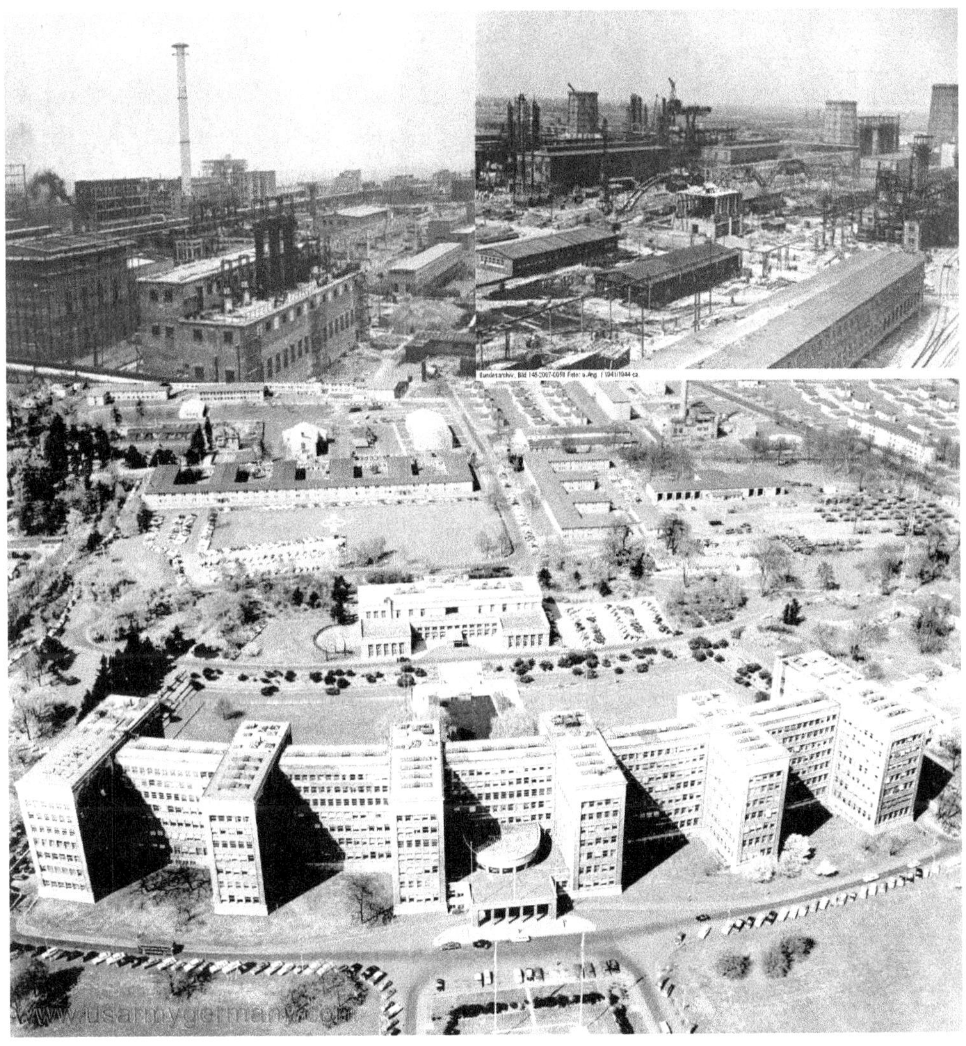

Do we understand by now how reality works? Charles Hingham's book, "Trading with the Enemy", gives extensive documentation of the Rockefeller activities during the Second World War. While Hitler's planes were dumping tons of bombs on London, they were spending money on royalties on gasoline they burned to Standard Oil, under existing patent agreements. After the war, Queen Elizabeth visited the US. She stayed in just one private home during her visit, the Kentucky estate of William Irish, of Standard Oil. Following the total destruction of most German cities from World War 2 air bombings, the I.G buildings remained intact by some miracle. The "dismantling" of I.G. Farben from 1945 to 1952 by the Allied Military Government, was a process similar to the "dismantling" of the Standard Oil empire by court edict in 1911. The Big Three created companies (Farben spin-offs) still behaved like a cartel. Who owns them all? Who owns Bayer for example?

The answer is the international banking cartel. In 1939, while it became clear that Germany would soon be unpopular in the United States, Standard Oil helped I.G. Farben cover its American holdings in the drug and chemical field. The American IG was formed, and transfer much of the finances to the US market by buying the Winthrop Chemical, Grasseli Chemical Works (alias the General Aniline Works), the Agfa-Film Company, the Sterling Products Company, and the Magnesium Development companies. Standard Oil received 15% of the stock in the new German-American chemical trust. Efforts to hook the DuPont corporation into this merger partially failed. Among the directors of the "cover-up" company were Walter Teagle (President of the Standard Oil Company), Paul Warburg (Rothschild agent) and Edsel Ford. The board of American I.G. had three managers from the Federal Reserve Bank of New York. American I.G. also had interlocks with Bank of Manhattan (later to become the Chase Manhattan), Ford Motor Company, Standard Oil of New Jersey, and A.E.G. (German General Electric). Three German not American members of the board of this American I.G. were found guilty at Nuremberg War Crimes Trials. Among these Germans was Max Ilgner, director of the I.G. Farben N.W. Seven offices in Berlin, i.e., the Nazi pre-war intelligence office. With the Pearl Harbor and US entering WW2 American IG Farben chose to cover its German origin and alliances, with the help of Standard Oil. It converted its name to the General Aniline & Film Corporation shortly before the Pearl Harbor attack. Before doing this, American IG bought an undisclosed number of shares in the Monsanto Chemical, Drug Incorporated, Mission Corporation, Dow Chemical, Schering & Company, Ozalid Corporation, Antidolar Company, Aluminum Corporation, Standard Oil of California, Standard Oil of Indiana, Standard Oil of New Jersey, and the DuPont Company. It took over Hoffman-LaRoche Company too. Under the Nazis, the German branch of chemical corporation and Standard Oil was simply a single firm. It was merged with hundreds of cartel arrangements.

I.G. Farben was led, up until 1937, by the Warburg family. Rockefeller's manager in the banking who helped design Nazi Germany eugenics and who was actually again just agent for Rothschild syndicate. Following the German attack on

Poland in 1939, Standard Oil promised to keep the merger with I.G. Farben going even if the U.S. joined the war. The merger was probably planned by Rothschild London banking cartel even before the war. Rockefellers by some extent was representing the interest of the Rothschild family on the other side of the Atlantic but underlining it is the same controlling force that financed all of this. When the American soldiers entered the manufacturing city of Frankfort, they remained amazed to discover the buildings in perfect condition and the huge plant of the German IG Farben Chemical Trust intact. American aviators completely demolished every other structure in town. Farben factory in Frankfort, one of the largest constructions there, miraculously remained intact. It was hardly accidental that the postwar government of Germany, Allied Military Government, also established its offices in the I.G. Farben building. This administration was headed by General Lucius Clay, who later became a partner of Lehman Brothers. What the doughboys also didn't know was that the Secretary of War, Robert P. Patterson, was a Rockefeller lawyer. He was appointed by President Roosevelt fresh out of Dillon, Read, and Company. The Dillon-Read company not only is a Rockefeller subsidiary but was the banking house that funded German IG Farben and tended to the commercial details of forming the American "cover up" firm for the German chemical cartel. In medicine, the Rockefeller cartel continues its medical monopoly. Control of the cancer industry is going through the Sloan Kettering Cancer Center. All of the major drug firms were funded from Chase Manhattan Bank, the Standard Oil Company or other Rockefeller firms. The American College of Surgeons keeps control of hospitals through the powerful Hospital Survey Committee, with members appointed by and for representing the Rockefeller control. On the other side of the Atlantic, it was the same thing.

Rockefeller that created his monopoly by coffins of National City Bank of Cleveland is not the independent individual. I only had been able to merely scratch the surface of the analyzing the all-pervasive influence of the Rockefellers and their foreign controllers, the Rothschild's, in every aspect of regular people lives. After November 1910, when Senator Nelson Aldrich chaired the secretive conference at Jekyll Island which gave rise to the Federal Reserve Act, the Rockefellers have kept the US inside the circle of the London Connection. After all of the consolidation, the now global medical industry cartel has been created. As planned. One monopoly of one medical and chemical industry that is part of a larger cartel of entire global international banking and financial system and military and other industry's consolidated into one controlling factor of enormous proportions that undermined the democratic process in the governmental level and undermined judiciary and everything else that can be undermined. And not just in the U.S. but on the global scale. Just not publicly but secretively. This system does not want you to learn for example the history of the creation of Big Pharma because they want you to watch the mainstream media and be good boys in school and go with the line. Government is there to protect you. Wars are there for peace and doctors are there to care for your health and health of your children.

If you make your opinion or assumption that some of the diagnosis or the treatment might not be valid to highly titled and highly ranked medical professional (professor, specialist, scientific researcher or adviser and so on), his psychological makeup will perceive it not just as personal attack but an attack on the entire of the science of medicine that backs him up. It is the medical branch that has authority just by itself to determent what health is and anything else to do with it. So when a doctor says something related to the health any layman opinion has no merit. From my personal experience the level of anger they can experience is high when I with my "uneducated" background begin to contradict their diagnosis and treatments and usually I am right and have in some cases more insight than them. That can be severely psychologically disturbing for some reason for their entire profession. Why? Because of the medical licensing. Medical license to do medicine creates fear for their future job security. It you contradict them they have a big problem because in their mind is the constant fear from liability. The psychological defense mechanism will be aggression. The doctors are educated to the highest standards, and we are not. They had spent six years just in college in learning, and we are not. They spend time in conventions and constantly learning to keep in touch with science, and we are not. And of course, it is widely known how much the medicine is a scientific field. Not everyone can do medicine. Only verified and educated person and that is it. Period. Do you have a problem with that? Well, there is the World Health Organization to make sure that you do not. It is exactly these two things that capitalism has brought into medicine: certification and qualification. The only question is who was the one that made the entire system of qualification (education)? In other words, who gives approval to some individual to do medicine. It is exactly what Rockefeller and his chemical-pharmaceutical cartel did. It is exactly what was systematically designed and pushed by a cartel from the beginning of the 20th century with the finish after the WW2 when medicine was socialized as a system of mass health care on the governmental level which include also the system of preventive medicine as well. And all of this is mandatory and in control of the state. Today your health and wellbeing is a concern of the state not your own. You are to do what state, school and media tell you to do and be a good citizen. It is a necessary mechanism (the law). However, there is one big secret and that is that state works with Big Pharma behind your back. Big Pharma is the one that is in charge and make all the money out of it. That was the intention of banking elite and their plan for new medical industry. To use the state as an enforcer.

They passed different laws one in 1939 known as: "The Wagner National Health Act." They used the already mentioned Robert Ferdinand Wagner, Rothschild agent from Germany to do so. Senator Wagner's bill, the National Health Act of 1939, provided overall support for a public health plan to be financed by federal grants to states and administered by states and localities. The Wagner Bill grew and turned from a proposal for federal grants-in-aid to a program for public health insurance. Originally launched in 1943, it shifted to Wagner-Murray-Dingell Bill. The bill asked for mandatory national health insurance and a payroll tax. The compulsory insurance. Exactly what they wanted the whole time. Resistance to this bill was gigantic, and the opponents started a brutal red-baiting assault on the board stating that one of its key policy analysts, I.S. Falk, was a conduit between the International Labor Organization (ILO) in Switzerland and the United States government. The ILO was red-baited as "an awesome political machine bent on world domination." Although the Wagner-Murray-Dingell Bill generated extensive national debates, with the intensified opposition, the bill never passed by Congress despite its reintroduction every session for 14 years! Had it passed, the Act would have established compulsory national health insurance funded by payroll taxes. You need to understand that the state is there as a smokescreen and enforcer of the secret agenda that is behind all of this. The agenda that you are not supposed to know or see. It has been done in most of the globe and industry still is going to push for more control. Your life is in not yours. Your life is theirs. It is in the hands of certified individuals. Visits to the doctor office have become something normal and mandatory in the life of every modern human being. People are indoctrinated into the belief that without the supervision of the doctors and checkups and vaccines and drugs we would all die or be deformed and that evading regular checkups is something primitive and dangerous. There is no life without the doctor's supervision, and the sad thing about it is that life is actually not their business at all. Quite the opposite.

Doctors where transformed into factory workers. By the new Rockefeller laws, they were employed and paid by the state. They were to do their eight-hour shift and get their pay no matter if they actually heal someone or not or if a patient died at their hands. By this new laws doctors where practically removed from the patients and put into the industry hands because they did not have any interest anymore to help anyone because they have their pay one way or the other. There are going to have the interest to not lose that pay by disobeying the industry guidelines and do things that are outside of prescribing drugs and surgery. And the pay was good. Doctors annual income begun to rise dramatically and they had become the elite profession becoming part of a middle and upper class. In past times that was not the case. However, we do not need to worry. If we just have any doubts, the governmental website Open Payments Data allows us to completely comprehend the economic connection between doctors and pharmaceutical companies in the United States. It does not need a high level of comprehension to understand what this is (emotional manipulation to ease your mind, marketing and propaganda by the government to get you back into the line), especially because it is rather a mystery that pharmaceutical corporations basically buy out the medical industry. It is unlikely that your own physician created the prevailing composition of the medical industry. Your physician may not even know the complexity of the pharmaceutical industry. Arnold Relman, Harvard Professor and former editor of the New England Journal of Medicine, described the situation flawlessly when he wrote: "The medical profession is being bought by the pharmaceutical industry, not only in terms of the practice of medicine but also in terms of teaching and research...The academic institutions of this country are allowing themselves to be the paid agents of the pharmaceutical industry. I think it is disgraceful."

Yes, but you might say that all of this is in the past. Today we have more democracy and freedoms with better governmental control and so on. The answer is no. We have even less freedoms then after WW2. We have been brainwashed in the schools and by the media infused with psychological research for social control, but nothing else is different. The same structure of control exists and have been existing from Middle Age and even before that. I will give one more recent example. You'd probably never heard that Bayer (IG Farben) paid tens of millions of dollars to end a three-decade-long scandal in which the company sold HIV-contaminated blood products to hemophiliacs, thousands of whom later died from AIDS. Bayer was eventually forced into signing checks to individuals that acquired AIDS because, in the 1980s, the Cutter Biological section of Bayer neglected federal law and recruited gay men with high risk and intravenous drug users, and prisoners as donors of the blood that Cutter later used to produce Factor VIII and IX. It is a drug, the clotting product, that hemophiliacs need in order to not bleed to death. In 1997 Bayer was sentenced to pay 300 million into a compensation fund for hemophiliacs with HIV. About 20,000 individuals caught HIV from the drug. Ironically, Bayer's new hemophilia iPhone app got some coverage, as did Bayer's hemophilia research grant to the University of Florida. On July 16, 1982, the United States Centers for Disease Control and Prevention (CDC) suggested that three hemophiliacs had acquired the AIDS. Epidemiologists began to think that the virus was spreading through hemophiliac's medication that they inject once every week. Medication was made from large pools of donated plasma from different people. Some of it was collected before mandatory HIV testing, often from homosexuals and drug users and in some prisons. Without an infection test, they had no way to determine does the plasma donors carried the virus. In January 1983, the manager of Bayer's Cutter Biological department confirmed in a letter that: "There is strong evidence to suggest that AIDS is passed on to other people through ... plasma products." These letters surfaced in trials and were found by some of the investigative journalists that later broke the story public. By May 1983, a Cutter competitor started producing a heat-treated concentrate that killed the virus, so France for example and many other countries decided to halt all clotting concentrate imports. Cutter worried losing consumers, so according to an enclosed memo: "Want to give the impression that we continue improving our product without telling them that soon we were also going to have a heat-treated concentrate." By June 1983, a Cutter letter to distributors to 20 countries said that: "AIDS has become the center of irrational response in many countries", and that: "This is of particular concern to us because of unsubstantiated speculations that certain blood products may transmit this syndrome." They lied, and many countries were still using the old concentrate. On February 1984, Cutter became the last of the four major blood product companies to get US approval to sell heated concentrate. They waited as long as possible. Still even after Cutter started to sell the new product, still for several more months, they continued making the old medicine. They just don't care. The reason was that the corporation had several fixed-price contracts and thought that the old product would be cheaper to produce. Bayer officials (responding on behalf of Cutter) responded with another lie: "Because some customers doubted the new drug's effectiveness, some nations were slow to support registration of new drug". Then they lied by telling that they had a shortage of plasma, that is used to make the medicine. For example, Taiwan was one country that still received the old HIV infected drug. Hsu Chien-wen, an official at Taiwan's health department, told in 2003 that Cutter had not appealed for approval to sell the heated medicine until July 1985. That was entire year and a half after doing so in the United States. In Hong Kong, for example, Cutter did not even need approval but only an import license in the 1980s to be able to import and sell the newer product in which normally takes one week. A company meeting notes that: "There is excess inventory." Because of already produced excess, company was resolving to: "Review international markets again to determine if more of this product can be sold." Because of the lack of control and corruption Cutter decided to dispose of stockpiles of older HIV positive drug to third world countries while selling the new, safer product in the West. If some of the people catch AIDS well, they can take aspirin for pain. And of course, this is all third world countries, so it is going to go well with eugenic programs of depopulation of the planet. When hemophiliacs in Hong Kong all of the sudden started to test positive for HIV, local physicians raised the question whether Cutter was dumping AIDS tainted medicine into less-developed countries. Cutter rejected the accusation, insisting that older drug had no severe hazard risk and was, in fact, the same fine product we have supplied for years. Hong Kong did not believe the lie, and when local distributor asked for the newer product, Cutter responded that all of the newer products was going to the US and Europe. For Hong Kong, and other third world countries they could make an exception for a small amount for the "most vocal patients." Meaning influential people that could potentially make a problem for them. So if you are a son of a politician, they will give you a safe new drug.

The United States Food and Drug Administration helped to keep the news out of the public eye. Government is not there to protect you and never had been. In May 1985, the FDA's regulator of blood products, Harry M. Meyer Jr., considering the companies had violated a voluntary arrangement to remove the old drug from the market, called directors of the corporations and directed them to comply. Cutter's internal notes from their meeting show that Meyer required that the issue is: "Quietly solved without alerting the Congress, the medical community and the public" and also noted that the FDA wanted the matter solved "quickly and quietly." Also at that time, Cutter official wrote that: "It appears there are no longer any markets in the Far East where we can expect to sell substantial quantities of nonheated-treated medicine." They sold the AIDS tainted medicine as long as possible with no empathy. The effects of all of this are impossible to calculate because there was no test for HIV, so we do not know how many people were infected with HIV before Cutter began selling its safer medicine or afterward. Cutter also sold the old medicine in Argentina, Indonesia, Japan, Malaysia, and Singapore after February 1984. Cutter shipped more than 100,000 vials of unheated concentrate, worth more than $4 million after it began selling the safer product. The sales continued partly because of Cutter's desire to deplete stocks of the older medicine, and partly because of fixed-price contracts, for which the company believed the older product would be cheaper to make. U.S. Justice Department had never investigated any corporate executives. Bayer in the past even marketed heroin for children. That is the level of psychopathic nature of these people.

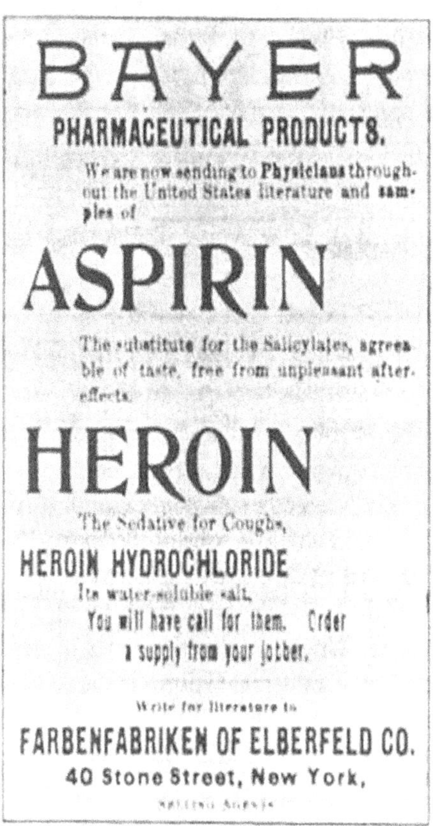

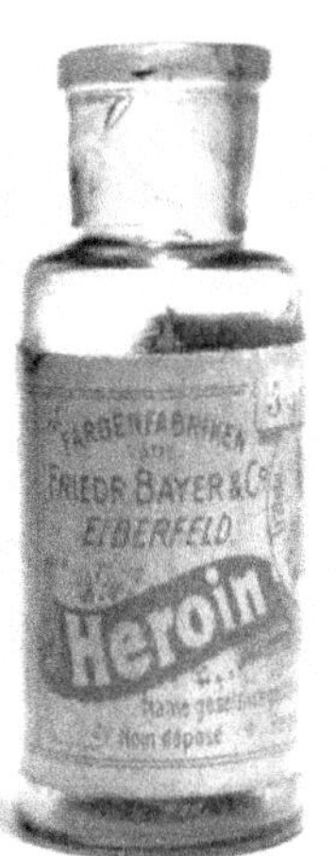

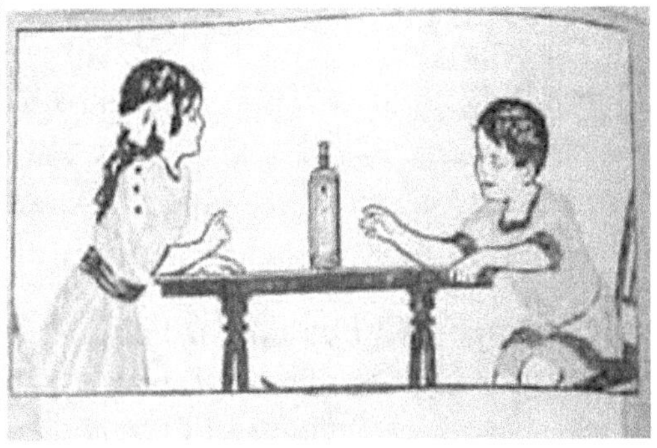

Now, do we think that this is all just in the past and that we live in the advanced democratic human rights granted world of equal opportunities painted by the mainstream media governmental propaganda? Let me ask this. If they actually researched and spend hundreds of billions of dollars they earn and really produced medications that actually cured people, how would they continue to profit off our illnesses? Or would they just treat symptoms and lie? And actually, so much more than just lie. They murdered people, destroyed people, waged war against anything that threatens them. Anything that they cannot control is a threat. Both in the form of nature or in the form of technology that cannot be patented or technology that can be patented but is not very profitable because it cures disease instead of treating the symptoms. These people know exactly what the game is all about and they are playing very well.

Anything that comes from nature, it cannot be patented. There are not interested in that. Everybody can grow a plant. That is a direct threat to industry interest. If there is a cure for some disease in the form of lifestyle changes, there are not interested in that. If there is some medicinal herb that works it must be destroyed. If it cannot be destroyed, then it has to be forbidden by law. You translate that into the real world of FDA approval, and we get no interest in research into not patented medicine and no interest in research of conventional patented medicine that will really help people in the long run. And of course, the destruction of all things that exist already and has been proven to help. The way they do that is by the FDA. You know that FDA says that it is illegal to use anything in existence unless it has been tested. You see the catch 22. Nothing from nature will ever be proven to be effective or safe because there is no one that is allowed to do the research and that has the money to do the test because there is no patent at the end of the test and no profit. They have control over you, and they do not like you. FDA does not do any testing of the drugs or supplements. It relayed solely on submission form the drug companies when it makes its approval. In any retrospective, it is designed to protect the industry, and it is the conflict of interest. It also has one more benefit for the industry. There is concern that the FDA has power now to remove from the marketplace all of the new dietary ingredients that were introduced after October 1994. This includes a big chunk of supplements that are on the market.

People can go and buy potent herb extras or other supplement and they can regulate their diet and lifestyle and get off the prescribed medicine, so the new law was passed in 1994. The FDA requires that manufacturers and distributors who wish to market dietary supplements that contain "new dietary ingredients" notify the FDA about these ingredients. Information requirement is to include information that is the basis on which the manufacturer or distributor has concluded that new dietary ingredient will reasonably be expected to be safe. What the safe actually means. In the first decade of the new dietary ingredients guidelines, the FDA took conservative view what dietary ingredient was. They will say that if it was in the food supply and if you can show that it is in the food supply then they will allow you to sell it and not require you to make a scientific submission. In the '90s FDA by the pressure from the industry took the more restrictive approach by expending the definition of a dietary ingredient and started to keep more things out of the market and is increasingly trying to regulate even the old supplements. The public reported purpose for the guidelines was to promote public safety for consumers. In reality, it had other intended purpose. Most of the supplement companies today were not present in 1994. Of those that existed hardly any had records. What FDA is saying now that your product is approved but only if you can scientifically prove it is safe because being on FDA published list before 94 is no proof anymore. So you have to do the studies, and that seems fine if you are not familiar with already mention catch 22. And of course, when the industry does their studies, they have billions to spent to alter the result in the desired way. We can only remember stories about aspartame and MSG approval. I will talk about it later in more detail. So today FDA basically require sort of preapproval from the companies and represent sort of economic barrier for entry. This will result in loss of small supplement manufactures and creation of small amount of big supplement companies that can be purchased by the Big Pharma and controlled. It cost somewhere in between from 150,000$ to about 1,3 million per one NDI (new dietary ingredients) submission. FDA also made the situation that approval of NDI is valid only for the company that submitted for it and it is cannot be transferred to any other company even if it is the same ingredient. Any human with a brain will understand just by this statement what FDA is doing and the scope of corruption. They require every company that sales the same ingredient to submit new dietary ingredient submission. As a result, there are now even fewer supplements and are even more expensive, and supplements that are pushed are the ones that are useless or dangerous but are in the industry interest to get pushed like protein powders and bodybuilding chemicals and so on. But if you want to buy for example curcumin extract as a support for cancer treatment then it will be more expensive than it should supposed to be and there was even push to force for example curcumin to be pharmaceutical prescribed as a drug, but it failed.

However, the intention is there, and it goes in one direction. If there was any way to ban the turmeric plant and many other plants they will gladly do it with no hesitation. Because there is not or it is hard to do because curcumin does not have any psychoactive properties and it is just a spice there is nothing that industry can do. However, then we have these forms of economic manipulations going on. Ingredients that we use to manage our health from foods to concentrated nutrients sold as dietary supplements are now being given requirements to prove safety before they can be used. Also it is hard to believe but they want to ban the medicinal foods too. The FDA Food Safety Modernization Act of 2007 (FSMA) gave the FDA unprecedented power over food. It gave the power to ban interstate commerce with any food in existence that have been studied for medicinal use. This act gives the FDA more power and more money to hire agents to run around the countryside of the USA to begin to arrest small organic gardeners, and to intimidate even people who grow food for themselves in their own yards and gardens.

The idea that you take some plant that is grown for millennia and require to enforce all kind of double-blind placebo studies that underlines regular drug testing is designed not to protect consumers but to remove the choice and to take responsibility for our own health from us and to put it in the hands of industry and its enforcer the government. And they did it already to the empirics and natural healers in the beginning of the 20th century but did not target individual people. Now they are going to target regular people as well. What are they going to do with this new authority is the same thing that they have done before. Every product that comes on the market would be assumed to be an unsafe product, any natural herb should be assumed to be dangerous, any other medical treatment not approved by the FDA should be assumed to be dangerous, every natural remedy, supplement or anything else if not approved should be assumed to be dangerous and are going to be removed until people manufacturing that product prove that the product is safe. And if a product is already proven to be safe, the approval needs to be done again for every single company. The small farmer who wants to sell medicinal herbs is going to be treated in a same way as selling dangerous substances for example like selling poisons or cannabis. It started to happen already today, but the intention is to be even more enforceable in the future.

By current law what agency can do to the small farmers or small companies that did not approve their products is that they can come and take everything farmer or company owns of any value. They can do it without any advance notice. Weapons drawn, barging into business seizure assets, freezing bank accounts, seize all the products, seize all the material inside the offices, computers, papers, files before trial or conviction. Charges can be both civil and criminal and can result in incarceration for a lifetime. Even if you don't get indicted, what they do is ruin someone business completely. They did start to do this to some extent to the local farmers especially in regards to raw milk and herbal remedies, but there was some backlash, but that did not stop the intention. What this in reality is all about is to start to push the small business out. If you have a small family supplement company can you afford to spend up to 1 million for approval for every product? What would you do most likely is to send your kid to college so that he can get a job at a regular pharmacy and close. It is not logical to conclude that government force companies to test one ingredient that has been proven to be safe over and over again just for safety and what is completely out of the scope of logic is to force payment that goes up to more than million dollars. The real intention is to economically burden and remove the small organic farmers and businesses, natural herbal doctors that are outside of the medical line and all other "threats" with this well-calculated economic warfare. And this is not just in the US. It has gone global. War on plants had been waged by industry monopolist for more than 100 years now, and the final chapter is already written in the UN. It is called Codex Alimentarius. That is fancy Latin name for the world food code. The ambiguous title "Codex Alimentarius" is no accident. It was written by the same companies and even in some cases the same individuals, who wrote the Auschwitz concentration camp slogan "Arbeit mach frei" ("Work makes you free"). It was created in 1963s in the UN by the same oligarchy. It is a body that was established by the Food and Agriculture Organization of the United Nations (FAO), and the World Health Organization (WHO). In fact, Codex is the next stage of intention for multi-national corporations razed above national sovereignty and enforced upon the world. The five segments of business that benefit from Codex are Big Bio-Tech, Big-Chem, Big Medica, Big Pharma, and Big Agra biz.

You will have a hard time accepting this but let's look again into the history of its creation. Fritz ter Meer, born in 1884, was a board member of IG Farben from 1925. Fritz ter Meer was the son of Edmund ter Meer (1852–1931), who established the chemical company Teerfarbenfabrik Dr. E. ter Meer & Cie in Uerdingen. This company was included in 1925 as a part of IG Farben. He was personally included in the preparation of Monowitz concentration camp.

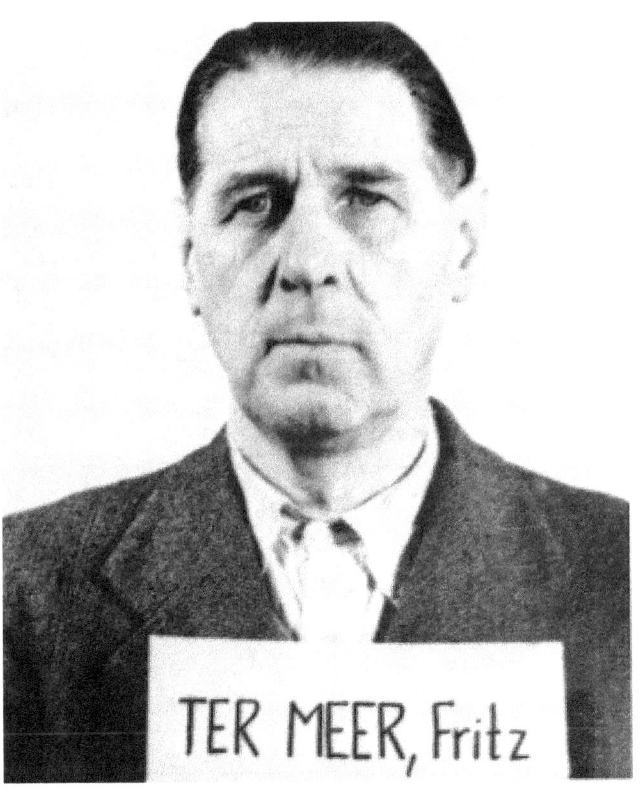

It was a new Auschwitz camp constructed for I.G. Farben. He was also responsible for helping build the IG Farben Buna Werke factory at Auschwitz, which conducted human experiments both for the war effort and for developing new drugs for IG Farben and held some 25,000 slave laborers under deplorable conditions. Meer was tried at the Nuremberg IG Farben Trial and was sentenced to seven years imprisonment. Which is nothing for the war crimes he was accused of and was involved. When he was questioned whether he had thought the tests on live people in Auschwitz are justified, he answered that this was irrelevant: "They were prisoners thus no particular harm was inflicted, as they would have been killed anyway." Well, no lies there but also a high level of psychopathy. Fritz ter Meer and twenty-six other I. G. Farben employers stayed strongly engaged in what the Germans called "the killing of useless eaters" or people who are alive but not deserving to live. They produced the compounds like the gas, Zyklon B, used to kill prisoners. However, you already by now know this. What you do not know is that during a time in prison, Fritz ter Meer theorized that using food as a weapon was the key to achieving world domination. He concluded that: "He who controls food, can control the world." He was right completely. By the guidance of Nelson Rockefeller, Fritz ter Meer's and all other sentenced IG Farben managers were "rescued" from jail already in 1952. Not only that, they had reassumed positions in the highest levels of German industry. After his release war criminal Fritz ter Meer was appointed yet again as a board member of Bayer in 1955 and, in 1956 was appointed a chairman of Bayer Pharmaceuticals. Like nothing had happened. He died in 1967 and what Bayer did? Bayer named student foundation after him. He had a plan forged in prison. He assembled all of the executives of former I. G. Farben, recommending a greater plan. They agreed and wrote the letter to urge the United Nations to take over the regulation of world food. Fifteen years after the Nuremberg War Crimes Tribunal they were planning world food domination as an act of population control. This actually happened.

The UN response was: "What a good idea." As a response to a letter and political pressure in 1962, the Codex Alimentarius Commission was formed. In 1963, already they started to create the standards and guidelines that are going to be obligatory in the future. They began to regulate everything that goes into your mouth: water, food, minerals or vitamins, or something else. If it goes into your mouth, then there is a standard for it. However, in reality, they have different agenda that is different from the public one of protecting the consumers. Codex, for example, allows pesticides, GMOs (genetically modified organisms), irradiation of food, and restricts supplements. For example, in July of 2007, the Codex committee on pesticides brought back seven from the nine banned and deadliest known pesticides in the world. The US is as I write this constructing 200 radiation plants to irradiate every bite of food so that the US can be in line with Codex guidelines. Here is one more example. FDA analysis and other studies have always shown that consumers do not like to buy genetically modified or irradiated food. The FDA to correct this false, unscientific opinion of stupid consumers wants to prevent the consumers from making the wrong choice. FDA believes that truthful labeling would be false and misleading.

Truth is false. That is Orwellian doublespeak. FDA believes that they know how to take care of you instead of you. Your life is in the hand of certified professionals. It is not your choice. In another word, Codex forbids labeling of GMO. You might don't know this but when you buy meat of any other product if it is GMO or irradiated you would not know that because there is no labeling. If you know how in reality the things are done and you know all the connections between the Rockefellers and the UN, as well as the common belief system of eugenics and population reduction, then you can understand the policies of eugenics that had been written in the architecture of Codex Alimentarius. The plans of a one-world global society built upon eugenics were not born with Adolph Hitler, and they certainly did not die with him. Codex, after all, is an organization created under the FAO and WHO, which are both under the jurisdiction of the UN. The connections between the pharmaceutical industry, medical establishments and their agenda pushed under the umbrella of the UN for the destruction of the natural healthcare industry, and natural supplement access is finishing blow in a war on plants that last for more than a 100 years now. The worst-case scenario for Codex Alimentarius, if it were to be implemented, is complete suppression of vitamin, mineral and other supplements.

How are they going to do is? They are going to decide what is standard and what can be produced. If they decide that RDA for some vitamins is out of the range, then that and any other supplement that has higher potency will be "dangerous for health" and will be forbidden for manufacturing and sales as a dangerous product. All of the high potency dietary supplements that we can buy today will no longer be on the market. What you would see are low potency supplements that don't do anything. Codex is going along with industry by pushing GMO, poisoning us with Melamine, poisoning us with Ractopamine led alone fluoride but have a big concern with overdosing on vitamins. The move by Codex to put maximum permissible limits on vitamins is what? What is it? Evil agenda or consumer protection? I am paranoid, so I know my answer. The levels they want are so small that they are below the line for prevention of chronic deficiency diseases. For example, I take around 5000 IU of vitamin D daily. The maximum level permitted by Codex is 10 IU. Ten. One more thing. If I believe that there are studies that had showed that amount of 5000 IU vitamin D daily is most beneficial I am not allowed to read them or have access to them because an official medical line is different and they have a concern that consumers will hurt themselves. Anything that is different from the medical line of accepted medicine is forbidden to be spread as health danger and hazard. Free speech is American fantasy a soon to be over. The Codex forbids this book for example. You as a consumer would never know what is going on and eventually you as uninformed individual will accept that yes 10 IU of vitamin D3 is a good thing. Anything above is illegal. I do not know about general public and general complacency with all of this but when I read Codex or other UN agendas like Agenda 21 all I see as a paranoid individual is the stuff of horrors. And this is just part of the prolonged war that had been going on for a long time now. Let us take a brief look at some examples in history of this war on plants or let say the war on health in general. And it is not just plants that are a problem because they cannot be patented. It is more than that. Every real cure that destroys the disease in its roots to never return is not something the industry wants even if it can be patented. They do not want cures they just want treatments that can prolong life a little. Let us look at real-life examples. They are the best for understanding how things work.

In a small town in Northern Ontario, back in 1922, rumors began circulating of some cancer-curing tea that was originating from the forests of Ontario. The Canadian Ojibwa tribe originally used a mixture. Indians called this mixture "tea of life." On a fateful day in 1922 Canadian cancer nurse, Rene Caisse noticed scar tissue on the breast of an elderly English woman. She was diagnosed with breast cancer 30 years before and that she cured it naturally without surgery. The woman did not have the money for it. She met an Indian medicine man who told her that in his tribe tradition they could cure the disease with some tea. She had nothing to lose. So she tried the tea, and it worked for her. She was still alive 30 years later when nurse Caissie examined her. She also told the ingredients of the herbal remedy to the nurse. Year after that nurse Caissie still didn't do anything with the tea she had heard about, but some local doctor in a walk told her that if the world uses some weed they walked by there will be no more breast cancer. It was the one of the weed in herbal remedy in that Indian medicine man tea. The weed was sheep sorrel. In 1924 she decided to test the tea on her aunt. Her aunt had nothing to lose because she had cancer of the stomach and conventional medicine at the time were given her about six months to live. She lived for another 21 years, cancer free. Rene Caisse (pronounced "Reen Case") later gave the tea to her 72-year old mother who was diagnosed with inoperable cancer of the liver, with only weeks to live. Her own mother healed and lived without cancer for another 18 years. After this events, Nurse Caisse decided to quit the hospital and began curing people with a mixture of herbs that would become known as Essiac which is her last name spelled backward.

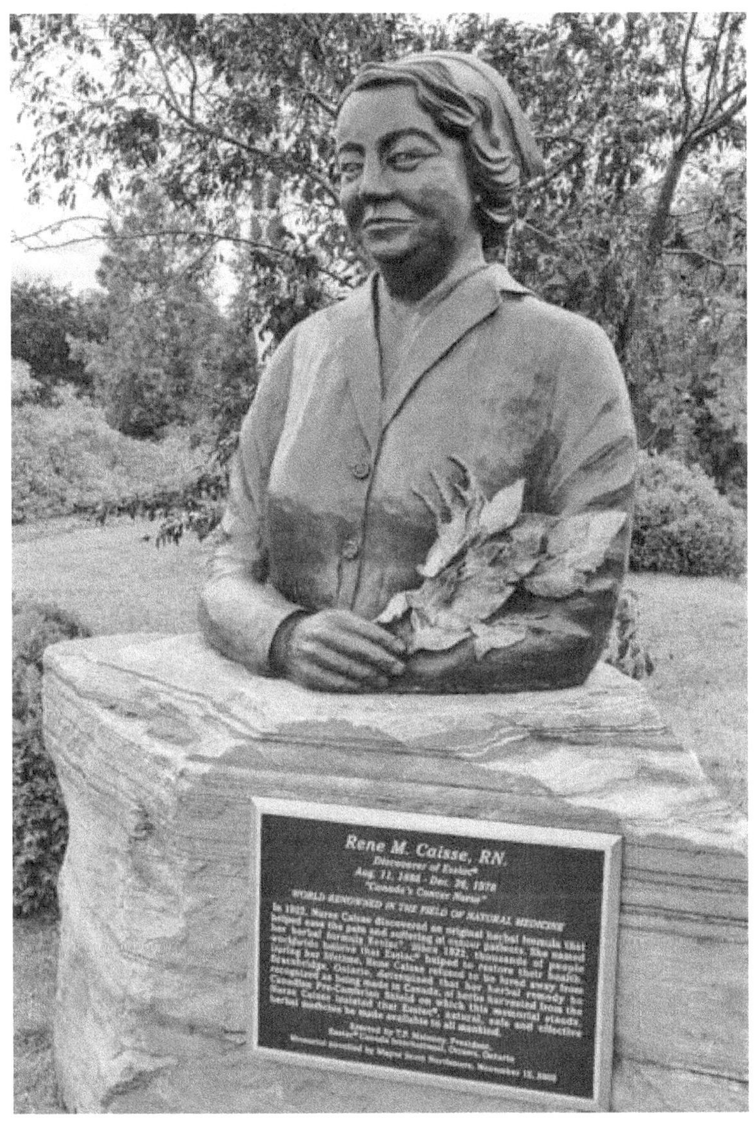

Soon the voice spread and a number of patients started to grow. When Dr. Bestida of Bracebridge, Ontario sent Cassie his patient Bert Rosin, and she cured him dr. Bestida went before town council and a mayor and persuaded them to give the Nurse Caisse the building as a clinic. They set up the clinic because Cassie made a great discovery and they wanted her to be supported by her own hometown. She treated for an eight and a half years there with patients flocking in from all directions. She treated around six hundred patients a week, and the only way she was allowed to do this is free of charge and she needed to have a doctor diagnosis for every case she treated. However, it was one Dr. Leonardo from Buffalo who had immediately recognized the potential of this cancer cure that warned her of what is going to happen. He was a cancer surgeon, and he asked if he can go to the clinic and examine patients to see for himself. After he had seen for himself, he sad to Cassie that she has it (the cure), but the medical profession will never going to let her do this. After a while of his visit, a small group mysterious "entrepreneurs" showed up offering Cassie a small sum of one million dollars for the secret formula. In that time one million was a big sum of money. The equivalent of 20 million today. Now we can think of this as a bribe to keep her quiet and go someplace warm and nice to retire. What tease "entrepreneurs" were not able to guarantee was that her cure would be made available for free or available at all to people that needed it. They just wanted the formula and her to go away. The only reason why we know about this today and you can read about it is because she refused. She was emotional and not pragmatic. She treated people for free in the clinic. Would you have refused such an offer? Who in her right mind would? How many other cures have been suppressed by this form of bribes that we do not know about, and we would never know?

In 1938 her case was called before the legislature to determent the Essiac legal status. She was trying to legalize her treatment. Her patients gathered 55,000 signatures for a petition. A bill was introduced in the Ontario legislature to: "Authorize Rene Caisse to practice medicine in the Province of Ontario in the treatment of cancer and conditions therein." Bill failed to pass. Public anger forced the establishment of a Cancer commission to investigate her remedies, but it was all rejected. Rene Caisse treated her patients under the supervision of many doctors. Some of those doctors saw with their own eyes what this tea could do, and eight of them signed a petition to the Department of National Health and Welfare at Ottawa, asking that Nurse Caisse be given facilities to do independent research on her discovery. Initially, Rene was not acquainted with the control that the medical/pharmaceutical industry had over governments. After the petition was delivered, she was continually threatened with arrest until she finally withdrew from public view. She kept on her clinic as long as she could until "they" stopped the doctors from giving the diagnosis and then she was forced to stop. Patients were still coming and in some cases begging her to treat them, but she was not able to do so without a diagnosis because she would be thrown in jail for a long time. She had a nervous breakdown and closed the clinic.

Essiac was cheap. Essiac is non-toxic. Essiac cannot be patented. She refused the bribe. In the normal world, such discovery would be welcomed with open hands and research would be done extensively to see what is the way of cancer suppression. In this world full of corruption stuff like this is labeled as fake and dangerous and in this case mass media owned by corporations could not demonize Nurse Cassie because she did not charge any money for the treatment.

They just quietly shot down the clinic and labeled it as a fake cancer cure that people should avoid without any research done. At that time, she had a diagnosis from the regular doctors. She had pathological findings and living patients in the thousands that were discharged from the regular hospitals and sent home to die. They went to her in the last stages of cancer and lived after the medical profession had given them up. And yet they refused to even acknowledge any benefits of the Essiac tea without even single research done. To this day The American Cancer Society states that: "Reviews of medical records of people who have been treated with Essiac do not support claims that this product helps people with cancer live longer or that it relieves their symptoms" and the FDA described Essiac as a "Fake Cancer 'Cure' Consumers Should Avoid." Cancer Research UK also remarks that: " There is no scientific evidence that Essiac can help to treat cancer or control its symptoms" and even warns that: "Essiac may interact with some types of cancer treatment, so it is very important to tell your doctor if you are thinking of taking Essiac."

After she recovered from the breakdown, she started again from scratch brewing the herbal mixture in her own basement and curing a small number of patients. Soon government began harassing her again and having her arrested more than once. But the story broke out, and JFK's personal physician, Dr. Charles Brusch who was also his close friend and who treated himself with Essiac when he battled cancer sent her invitation to test Essiac scientifically. Caisse gave some samples of Essiac to Dr. Charles Brusch, who was also the founder of the Brusch Medical Center in Cambridge, Massachusetts, where tests where done. This first scientific tests showed that Essiac is not toxic and did have positive effects on a cancer suppression. At that time Dr. Brusch recommended that Essiac should be tested for toxicity in order to be approved by the FDA as a possible cancer treatment. Once that tea arrived at the Sloan-Kettering Cancer Center process somehow got bogged down. A laboratory at Memorial Sloan-Kettering Cancer Center did test Essiac samples (provided by Caisse) on mice during the 1970s. This study was never formally published. There is controversy regarding the results. There were unexplainable delays, and more delays and process never got to any conclusion. Sloan-Kettering Cancer Center is supposedly one of the most important cancer research centers in the US. Chester Stock the Co-director of Sloan-Kettering, when interviewed by the news agency, said that: "Results that he reported showed that there was very small percentage in the small group of regressions, but they never had the opportunity to confirm this and to see whether they could obtain better results."

So in the end, Essiac was not approved by the FDA. Caisse refused offers by researchers at Memorial Sloan-Kettering and the U.S. National Cancer Institute for access to the recipe. It went so far that patients themselves started to organize for suing the government and FDA on couple occasions. They believed that under the constitution they could put in themselves any substance that they want as long as they are no danger to others and that no FDA or anybody else can tell them what they can or cannot use in their own body, so various groups of patients organized and sued FDA for denying them a possible cure. Court hearings went nowhere, and yes constitutional rights had been denied to them. Dr. Frederick Banting, the co-discoverer of insulin became interested in Essiac too and even offered Nurse Caisse research facilities to test it further, but by this time Rene had already lost her will to fight. The single woman Rene Caisse trusted to help her make Essiac tea was her best friend, Mary McPherson. According to Dr. Gary Glum, Mary had promised Rene never to share the recipe with anyone. It was one Dr. Glum that in 1985 purchased the formula for $120,000 from one of Rene's former patients. Dr. Glum could have kept the formula secret and become very wealthy selling bottles of Essiac. However, he unselfishly released the formula into the public domain in 1988. At first, he offered the formula on a videotape that he advertised in his book, but the feds unlawfully seized the tapes before he could sell very many of them. Dr. Glum gave out the Essiac formula and recipe free of charge to anyone who mailed him a request for the Essiac formula. When Dr. Glum met Mary McPherson in Bracebridge, Ontario and told her what the Essiac formula was, she was more than a little surprised. According to Dr. Glum, Mary eventually revealed the formula in 1994 because it was no longer a secret, and she wanted to end the controversy over the Essiac formula before she died.

Therefore, on December 23, 1994, the "Essiac" formula & recipe was officially entered into the public domain with the recording of Mary McPherson's affidavit. Essiac includes a mixture of different herbs, including sheep sorrel (Rumex acetosella), later proven to be the most potent one. Then also slippery elm inner bark (Ulmus fulva), burdock root (Arctium lappa) and Turkish rhubarb (Rheum palmatum). Slippery elm is the only Essiac herb native to North America. Turkey rhubarb (Rheum palmatum) is native to China and Tibet, not northern Ontario, so it appears unlikely that it was a part of the original medicine man's formula of indigenous herbs in the late 1800s. It appears that both burdock and sheep sorrel were brought to this continent from Europe by early settlers who then passed on their knowledge of these two herbs to the local tribes. Burdock and sheep sorrel eventually spread throughout North America where water was sufficient. Rene Caisse indicated that sheep sorrel was one of the original herbs, so it appears that sheep sorrel had migrated to the wilds of Northern Ontario before the 1890s. Burdock could have also established itself in Northern Ontario by then. René Caisse felt sheep sorrel was the most active cancer fighter among all the herbs present in her formula. Dr. Chester Stock shared that viewpoint at Sloan-Kettering. Dr. Stock conducted some studies on sheep sorrel benefits for over three years in the mid-seventies.

In 2012, there was one study done in Hungary. The results of a study out of Hungary were published and showed that the Sheep Sorrel herb, and a number of its Sorrel relatives, demonstrated substantial cell growth inhibitory activity (at least 50% inhibition of cell proliferation) against one or more cancerous cell lines. Score one for the herbalists. A survey carried in the year 2000 found approximately 15% of Canadian women with breast cancer to be using Essiac. It has also become popular in people with immune diseases such as HIV and diabetes and as a regular herbal tea as well as preventative measure in health-oriented individuals. Research conducted since Caisse's death provided some insight. Herbs used in making Essiac possess antioxidant and anti-cancer properties, according to research conducted at the European Institute of Oncology. The findings were reported in the March 2006 issue of the Journal of Ethnopharmacology. Researchers found that four of the herbs in Essiac demonstrated natural powers of protection against cancer. Finally, a quick search of PubMed archive can give us a couple of studies like (Inhibition of prostate cancer-cell proliferation by Essiac J Altern Complement Med. 2004 Aug;10(4):687-91). They examined cancerous cell line and spleen cells in vitro that had been isolated from mice to examine proliferation responses mediated by the addition of an Essiac. They found decreased proliferation of both noncancerous transformed and cancerous prostate cell line when Essiac was present in the culture media. That means that tea had stopped all cells from dividing, but the percent inhibition of the cancer cells was higher than the percent inhibition of the regular cells implying that Essiac may have an additional selective effect on cancer cells. On top of that, the effects of Essiac were measured in an immune T-lymphocyte proliferation assay. At low doses of Essiac, an increase of the proliferation of these T cells was demonstrated, but at higher doses, Essiac was inhibitory to T-cell proliferation. This means that Essiac may be able to inhibit tumor cell growth while enhancing the immune response. This may be particularly important in immune-suppressed individuals. Like in HIV. In this study (In vitro analysis of the herbal compound Essiac. Anticancer Res. 2007 Nov-Dec;27(6B):3875-82.) Essiac exhibited significant antioxidant activity, exhibited significant immunomodulatory effects, specifically through stimulation of granulocyte phagocytosis and moderately inhibiting inflammatory pathways. Essiac exhibited significant cell-specific cytotoxicity towards ovarian epithelial carcinoma cells (meaning it kills cancer). They concluded that this study was the first comprehensive investigation of the in vitro effects of Essiac and that in vitro analysis of Essiac indicates significant antioxidant and immunomodulatory properties, as well as neoplastic cell (a cell that is part of tumor) specific cytotoxicity (specific to killing only cancer cell) which is consistent with the historical properties ascribed to this compound. There are also other studies that did not find anything and even one study that finds increased risk of breast cancer (Essiac and Flor-Essence herbal tonics stimulate the in vitro growth of human breast cancer cells. Breast Cancer Res Treat. 2006 Aug;98(3):249-59. Epub 2006 Mar 16.).

So again we have conflicting science. Hundred years since the Essiac first appeared we still do not have a clear picture. In the world where supposedly there are hundreds of millions of dollars of cancer research spending annually (the reason why all of this cancer drugs supposedly cost so much) somehow it is hard to do a simple tea examination and research. Or any other examination for "alternative" cures for that matter. What FDA response is that the reason why they do not test these is that they do not want to give quacks the credibility. And they are lying. They do not want to give the "alternatives" any chance to prove their efficacy because they are not there to protect you or heal you. They are there to protect the Rockefellers Big Pharma business. There are many cases to be cited concerning congressional investigations I just used Essiac as one example. If you want you can go and read 1963 hearings of Senator Paul Douglas of Illinois on Krebiozen. The story goes something like this.

In 1944, a Yugoslavian refugee doctor, Dr. Stevan Durovic, a former assistant professor at the University of Belgrade established the Instituto Biologica Duga in Buenos Aires. He observed that horses with neck tumors caused by a fungus often died, but some would recover. He theorized that the survivors must have a better immune system that produces some substance that helped them overcome the disease. He experimented and allegedly came up with a process for extracting that substance. It was tested allegedly in dogs with great success. In 1949 an Argentine businessman Loretani introduced Dr. Durovic to two other businessmen, Ed Moore, and Kenneth Brainard, who proposed an idea for Durovic to go to the USA and meet with Dr. Ivy. Dr. Andrew C. Ivy, a was a medical researcher of impregnable reputation and gigantic stature in his profession. Dr. Ivy was vice president of the University of Illinois, head of its huge Medical School, Executive Director of the National Advisory Cancer Council, and he was also a director of the American Cancer Society. An important, a respected, an honored man and the man that will be hard to name as a quack.

So in 1949, he brought to the United States a substance named Kositerin (not Krebiozen), apparently beneficial in the therapy of hypertension. He contacted in Chicago, Dr. Roscoe Miller of Northwestern University. He intended that Kositerin is tested in high blood pressure patients. Presumably, test for that substance was negative. Later, Dr. Miller introduced Dr. Durovic to Dr. Andrew Ivy. Having come with Kositerin for hypertension, Dr. Durovic just happened to have available for him also the 2000 mg of material he stated came from the blood of horses that had been inoculated with Actinomyces bovis that showed good result in fighting cancer. Dr. Ivy found the idea attractive. Idea fitted with the views he held on chemical substances that must be present in the body to control the growth of tumors. Indeed, that basic concept that there must be internal control of growth of tumors by the immune system is shared by many and proven to be correct by research. The immune system does have some ability to fight cancer cells, and we all have cancer cell all the time just our immune system is good enough to keep them in control. Dr. Ivy became interested in the theory shown by Dr. Durovic's substance. He decided to test it in a scientific manner. The results were positive supposedly.

Though Krebiozen was used only on individuals who had been diagnosed as hopeless and close to death, and because of many controversies surrounding the case, we today cannot know what real effect this drug had if any. Allegedly there was a lessening or complete disappearance of pain, and in many cases, tumors were dissolved and replaced with healthy tissue. Dr. Ivy testified at his trial that without repeating the experiments, without previously having heard of Dr. Durovic as a scientist, without having seen analyses or manufacturing records or without knowing what was in the ampules, except for Dr. Durovic's word, he proceeded. After first injecting himself, Dr. Krasnow, and one dog, and without occurring to him (he testified) that the alleged substance X might be a hoax, Dr. Ivy injected the first patient on August 20, 1949. Colleagues and physicians continued the clinical trial. In 1951, Dr. Ivy after the research had been done chose to publish his findings. There was a press conference held in the Drake Hotel. It was a closed conference where the science writers of four Chicago papers, the Mayor of Chicago, two United States Senators, and potential financial supporters were invited, in addition to some physicians. Dr. Ivy testified that after testing on 22 patients and seeing beneficial results in 70%, a small private meeting was to be held at the Drake Hotel in Chicago. In his words, the idea was to find other scientists and clinics who would further the research effort. Eighty cancer specialists and doctors, four respected medical journalists were invited. Unfortunately, in public was sent out an unauthorized, sensationalist press release talking about patients who had been cured of cancer. Allegedly Dr. Ivy was horrified, but that did not change the fact that it was more in the line of marketing campaign business gathering then real scientific meeting. Results on 22 patients were presented. Of the 22, eight were dead, according to the table in a booklet distributed at the meeting, but is not a single instance was cancer listed as the cause of death. In each of the eight instances, however, as was brought out at the trial, the patients died with and of cancer.

Furthermore, two more of the 22 patients had died, one seven days and one two days before the meeting, both from cancer. The description in summary still stood as: "Dramatically clinical improvement. Now working all day without opiates. The patient had to be carried, couldn't walk." Over the ensuing years, there were lots of patients treated with Krebiozen. In the report on Krebiozen 79.5% of doctors who did try Krebiozen have been discouraged after a single patient. They only treated one. Ninety-two percent treated no more than two patients. The Krebiozen Research Foundation, however, claimed objective improvement with a decrease in tumor size in 61% of tumors of the brain and spinal cord, 70% of metastases to the brain, 48% of breast cancers. Three cases will later suffice to indicate the glaring inadequacy of critical assessment of patient records by the Krebiozen Research Foundation, but at the end of the day, this substance is not relevant at all. What is important is to understand the system and that is why I use this story as an example. With such merchandise as a cancer cure, humanitarian considerations are joined by the power, influence, and control. It is highly likely that powers at high places influenced by the reputation of Dr. Ivy believed that he actually did have something and were alarmed and decided to act. This is why two Chicago businessmen tried to get control of the distribution rights to Krebiozen. Same as Essiac same as any other story. They offer the bribe if not you are done. When they were refused, they threatened to ruin Krebiozen and everyone connected with it. One of the men who made this threat was the friend of J. J. Moore, the treasurer of the American Medical Association.

Even by February 1950 already the Moore and Brainard were demanding the distribution rights to the drug, but Dr. Durovic felt it was not proper because of their lack of expertise in this field and they were offered a royalty or partnership, but they reportedly refused all alternatives. AMA officials, Dr. Wermer and Dr. Moore, visited Dr. Durovic. At one point reportedly they said to him: "Don't you think you have an obligation to Moore and Brainard for the distribution rights to Krebiozen? You must give the distribution rights to Moore and Brainard." All of this was written in sworn testimony a year later, and you can do your own investigation. Testimony is publicly still available. Later in 1951, Loretani, who was a businessman from Argentina, met with the Durovic again. He made perfectly clear that:" If they did not get what they demanded, his powerful friend Dr. Moore would see that they, Dr. Ivy and their discovery Krebiozen would be utterly destroyed." Loretani told Durovic that Ed Moore had a good connection in the University of Illinois who would make an unfavorable report on Krebiozen. They were willing to hand over $2.5 million, and then all attacks would cease. In a meeting between Pick and Wermer, the Pick testified that he was told: "It is too bad a man of your caliber has to go down with the ship, but that is the way it has to be." In October 1951, The

AMA's study on Krebiozen was written in only six weeks. Usually, it takes two years or more for such a study. It was done on 100 patients of whom 98 showed no evidence of improvement. A few weeks later Dr. Ivy was put on trial by the Executive Committee of the Chicago Medical Society for breaking medical ethics and was suspended. This forced him to resign from all his medical posts.

Soon after that, the National Research Council wrote a letter published in the AMA Journal which said:" There was no proof of palliative effect attributable to Krebiozen". So far so good and this story would be forgotten by now. However, Commodore Barreira, who had been looking after Dr. Durovic's laboratory in Buenos Aires, was skeptical of the negative AMA report. He made a plan. He with his secretary acquired a meeting with Dr. J.J. Moore, the AMA operative. The plan was that Barreira pretended to have had a falling out with Dr. Durovic and to possess documents that were incriminating against him. Trusting Barreira's story, Dr. Moore, keen to get hold of these documents revealed AMA conspiracy for obtaining distribution rights to the drug. He even invited Mr. Barreira to became a partner in the scheme and affirmed to him the AMA would maintain its pressure until Durovic was overpowered and forced to sell out for scrap. Then, the plotters behind the AMA as rightful owners of Krebiozen would share the millions the drug was worth. Dr. Moore further said Dr. Ivy remained unreasonable in defense of Krebiozen. The conspirators had made him expelled from the Chicago Medical Society, and are going to have him turned out of his office at the University of Illinois. Mr. Barreira now had proof of all of the corruption and conspiracy. The conspiracy was discovered in the highest level of AMA, and with this proof, Barreira influenced the Illinois legislature to proceeded with the investigation. Hearings opened in April 1953. Commodore Barreira gave his affidavits and testimony. The AMA during investigation and afterword have never denied the action of their Treasurer. So did Dr. Moore himself. Reread this sentence again. The AMA has never denied the action of their Treasurer nor did Dr. Moore himself. You want proof of a deep state. Here you have it. Dr. Ivy destroyed the AMA Status Report, using words such as deception, falsification, misleading, unethical and fakery. The Hearings ended nearly a year later. They reported that Dr. Ivy's research had been conducted according to necessary scientific standards.

There were never make any conspiracy charges against Dr. Moore because their remit only pertained to the goings on at the University. Reread this again. The legislators never did make any, zero, no what so ever conspiracy charges against Dr. Moore because their remit only concerned to the goings on at the University and that is a lie. They did not because that would prove the criminal conspiracy at the level of American government involving an entire medical system of the

USA. Unfortunately, the Hearings appeared to change nothing. Later instead of going to jail, they voted Dr. Moore back in as Treasurer.

The National Cancer Institute declined to examine Krebiozen. Dr. Ivy's position as Vice President of the University of Illinois was not renewed. All of the medical and other journals rejected to write his research papers. The community was very excited about Krebiozen, and individuals who know about the drug some time asked their doctors to use the drug. However, all the studies show that it had no positive effect and there were reports from hospitals that they tested it and that it was worthless. One doctor from Sloan Kettering Memorial Hospital, New York, even wrote in a letter that: "We tried it on 100 patients". The only problem was that it was later found to be a lie. Some doctors also reported that their patients had died after using Krebiozen. The FDA supposedly did its own research, and the finding was that Krebiozen was only creatine, and then announced plans to prosecute Dr. Ivy and Dr. Durovic. Again the only problem was that in an actual trial that followed, FDA experts admitted they were "mistaken." Today at any official place we would find that Krebiozen was just creatine, but again it was proven to be a "mistake." In this case, you can see the scope of corruption. It was not a mistake, it was an organized effort for gaining or maintaining the control of the medical industry. When FDA experts admitted, they were mistaken that part of the sentence you would not read on Wikipedia. That part has been forgotten.

If it seems impossible that a "distinguished" cancer center would lie, please remember that Sloan Kettering was caught red-handed lying about different cancer therapy, Laetrile, and was exposed by one of its own employees, Dr. Ralph Moss, who was unwilling to participate in the fraud. The details of correspondence between three Sloan-Kettering cancer specialists and a Mrs. Dorothea Seeber on behalf of a friend in the last stages of cancer are one typical example. Sloan-Kettering doctors and their view of Krebiozen can be seen in a letter they sent to people who ask about it and whether it would be advisable to use it on a "hopeless case." "We tried it (Krebiozen) on 100 patients, and I regret to say that we could not substantiate any of the claims ascribed to its use." "I have had only a few patients who have been tried on Krebiozen, and there was no improvement in their condition." A third wrote: "A considerable amount of work has been done on this drug and we found it is absolutely worthless." An affidavit by Dr. Ivy tells a different story in which under oath you can read that he never provided or that these three doctors even ever received any of the drug. Until the date of the affidavit, not one ampoule of Krebiozen had ever been sent to the Sloan-Kettering Institute. Then the new FDA laws came into effect in June 1963, which meant that Krebiozen could not be sent over state lines without FDA approval, and of course, they had no intention of ever granting.

So, the substance could only be purchased in Illinois until 1973 when it was outlawed in Illinois too. The dealings that come out in public associated with this story is of dramatic proportions. There are falsified medical reports, South American undercover agents, threats of deportation, monitored phone calls and charges of influence by the Vatican. To illustrate this a reporter on the staff of the New York Post, called the AMA for specific answers to specific questions, such as: "Does J. J. Moore deny that he formed a conspiracy to gain control of Krebiozen?" Also: "Does the AMA deny that its official report against Krebiozen was falsified?" He was only met with this stock answer: "The AMA will not answer specific questions concerning Krebiozen." The reporter's s comment was: "It sounds a bit like the AMA is pleading the Fifth Amendment."

Krebiozen was just another unproven probably ineffective treatment, but that is irrelevant. Powers at be did not care and saw it just as another threat to their control. It is completely irrelevant what that drug was or was it effective. This case had proven in the court of law and also in the congressional hearings the true nature of medical and governmental corrupted reality, and if you do not want to see it, then that is your choice. If you have done much reading about alternative cancer treatments, you are aware there are a great number of therapies with stories similar to this. And that is just the ones that we know about. What would have happened if they decided to take the 2.5 million? They were greedy like any other doctors out there, and they thought that they could get much more out of it, but they underestimated and probably didn't understand the level of corruption. Cancer quackery is lucrative. Dr. Stevan Durovic was under indictment for evasion of income tax in the amount of $904,907 for the years 1960, 1961, and 1962 alone. Government investigators had shown at his trial that large sums of money were withdrawn from the bank accounts of the Promak Laboratory, money derived from the sale of Krebiozen and sent to Canadian and Swiss banks. However, Dr. Durovic did manage to get out. Or was allowed to. He told a Chicago reporter that he had flown nonstop from Chicago to London and then traveled to Paris. Internal Revenue agents told a Washington correspondent, however, that Durovic had flown from Miami to Bimini in the Bahamas, from Bimini to Nassau, from Nassau to Bermuda, and from Bermuda to London and from London to Paris. One of Durovic's attorneys has even filed a suit seeking $11,787 in unpaid legal fees. The problem here is how many other people did find something similar that actually did work against cancer but decided that they would take the bribe and go away peacefully. That is a rational choice. I would say nine out of ten. For every Krebiozen that we know there is nine other that are suppressed and never heard about. And the list of suppressing cancer therapies that were never tested by the FDA that we do know about is very long. If average person would go thru litany and read all at the congressional investigations looking into cancer and read 1963 hearings on Krebiozen or for example 1981 hearings of Senator Paula Hawkins from Florida that was investigating the fraud in the National Cancer Institute I think that it would be a lot of anger and emotions and uproar.

In 1986 an uproar of the cancer patients forced Congress to look into yet another one of the charges of medical suppression. The pattern was the same. Cancer researcher Lawrence Burton, Ph.D., had a successful cancer treatment by Immuno-augmentative therapy (IAT) that was developed by him. He claimed that it could control all forms of cancer by restoring natural immune defenses. A form of vaccination line therapy for tumors where the immune system is trained to recognize the tumor. He was injecting blood serum proteins isolated with processes he had patented. Dr. Burton's activity focused on cytokines. These are proteins that produce cell signaling functions inside the immune system. Some of these were later called TNF. He discovered that these could kill the tumor initially, but in time they stop to work. Dr. Burton theory was that to avoid toxicity in the body something must block TNF from attacking the tumor. He theorized that there must be a blocking protein. He thought that if he could eliminate the blocking protein, TNF would be capable of attacking cancer. He analyzed more than 3000 patients with a conclusion that cancer patients have a distinct profile which involves too little of unblocking protein, and too much-blocking protein. In his theory, to test it he every day took a small amount of blood from the subjects to measure different immune factors. Many blood plasma shots from donors are given throughout the day to balance the proteins. The process has been shown to extend the lives of many patients with advanced disease considerably and to give them an enhanced quality of life. However, Burton did not publish detailed clinical reports, divulge the details of his methods, published meaningful statistics, conduct a controlled trial, or provide independent investigators with specimens of his treatment materials for analysis. He constantly accused a government that it wants to get hold of his work and was a bit paranoid. However, he was probably right, and the pattern proved to be the same. National Cancer Institute accused him of quackery and refused investigation. If you ask the American Cancer Society, the existence of blocking and deblocking proteins has not been verified, and IAT is an unproven treatment. However, today we know that this treatment is more effective than any other treatment for some specific forms of cancer. Not for all but for some it is extremely useful. For example, treatment is a success with mesothelioma — cancer caused by asbestos. For this form of cancer, response if better than any other known therapy in the world or it can be used as an addendum to traditional treatments. However, it does not matter. He did not want to sell.

Burton later charged the NCI of illegally trying to attain his methods. They came after him like they always do so under pressure he moved his clinic to the

Bahamas in the 1970s. And It should also be noted that it was through Dr. Burton's research that TNF (Tumor Necrosis Factor) was discovered. He was not a quack. Dr. Lawrence Burton developed a system that could attack tumors in the early sixties. At the early stages of research, he got funding (The Damon Runyon Fund). The American Cancer Society sent him someone to work with him. Over the next two years, Dr. Burton's research flourished and expanded. Invited by the American Cancer Society to a national seminar of oncologists he did demonstrate his methods. In 1965, Burton did experiments in mice with solid tumors. It was observed by the American Cancer Society science editor himself, and he was shocked by what he saw. He reported: "They injected the mice, and the lumps went down before your eyes – something I never believed possible." The following year in 1966, under the American Cancer Society. Dr. Burton appeared before the New York Academy of Sciences and performed a demonstration in front of 70 scientists and 200 science writers. Mice were vaccinated with the serum, and ninety minutes later, the tumors had nearly disappeared basically before your own eyes and all of this in front of 70 scientists. Allegedly. Sounds too good to be true. Newspapers throughout the world ran the story on their front pages while the prestigious peer journals got their story from an investigator for Sloan-Kettering and Dr. Castle from the American Cancer Society. The Los Angeles Examiner wrote "Fifteen Minute Cancer Cure for Mice: Humans Next?". Philadelphia Bulletin: "Demonstrated before our very eyes that injection of a mysterious serum…caused the disappearance of massive tumors in mice within a few hours." However, the real cure is not what they want, so the medical community did not approve. They challenged the validity of the trial and advised that it has to be done by some trickery. Five top scientists were so enraged they organized a press conference. However, they were persuaded by their colleagues to cancel it. Later that year Dr. Burton and his associate Dr. Friedman were invited by the New York Academy of Medicine to repeat the experiment. This time, of sixteen mice with cancer on display, the gathered assembly of oncologists and pathologists chose which of them should be injected with the tumor-inhibiting factors. To avoid magic tricks neither Dr. Burton nor Dr. Friedman gave the serum. The result was the same as in the previous experiment. Again too good to be true. However, their precautions made no difference, as yet again he was accused of faking the whole experiment.

Then the contract negotiations came. The big wigs, NCI, Sloan-Kettering, American Cancer Society wanted to buy it up from Burton. They would give him grants and credit for it, but they wanted the rights. Burton turned them down. Burton became the enemy. The funding stopped. Invitations to speak vanished. Publications refused to publish. The attacks began. After he moved his clinic, he probably thought that he was safe, but his problems did not end there. It was successful therapy and a threat to the system of control. He and his clinic had to go no matter if they are not on the territory under control of American government directly. In 1985 the CNN and all other government control propaganda lunch the campaign against the clinic. Burton's serum came from human blood. So in 1985, in a speech by the Deputy Director of the National Cancer Institute, it was mentioned as if in an aside, that Burton's IAT specimens contained HIV. Supposedly two families returning from his clinic to US had brought back 18 sealed IAT specimens. A Washington State blood bank examined them, and all of them contained hepatitis B while some tested positive for HIV. The Bahamian Ministry of Health and Pan American Health Organization visited Burton's clinic, and in July of 1985, the Bahamian Government closed the clinic. Burton reopened his clinic in March of the following year, but in July, the FDA issued an import ban prohibiting anyone from bringing IAT into the United States. This ban is still in effect. And guess what, the congressional committee has since made these findings: "IAT Clinic was closed in July 1985 based upon a false and alarming claim spread by NCI personnel of an aids risk ". They concluded that the contamination report was false. It came from high NCI official. The inaccurate report was circulated in the AMA Journal, the officials from the White House and State Department. Even the families who had brought back sealed IAT specimens into the US never contracted hepatitis B nor were they ever tested to be HIV positive.

The closure of the Clinic accidentally coincided with the US releasing new drugs strikingly similar to the Burton one like Interleukin-2. As a result, 38 congressmen signed the formal request for the independent federal evaluation of "alternative" cancer therapies. The reality is that there is premeditated, well organized, global conspiracy to control and to maintain the status quo.

Conspiracy to prevent any threat to the system of control like finding the cure or "alternative" non-patentable therapies or mechanisms that could not be regulated by the institutions. The system includes FDA, Federal Government, parts of Congress, Big pharma and so on. The way of business has been established, and they are not going to let anyone from the outside to threaten their inner club. When I did my initial research into medical suppression, I did not think I would find much. What I did find didn't surprise me but what surprised me is the sheer number of cases. It is not just a couple of them. I stop my research at about 15. I lost the will. What surprised me is that in the era of information technology there is no real discussion or knowledge about this in society. It is not that one percent of psychopaths that run this show are doing what they are doing, it is surprising that the rest of 99% of the population is docile. The information is available, but there is a low level of understanding. Freedom of information is freedom of choice. If this course of business continues in the near future, the information itself will be suppressed.

The worst case of medical suppression in entire human history was the case of suppression of what I like to call broad specter resonance radiation technology (BSRR) first invented by Dr. Royal Raymond Rife. He did not name his invention this way. There was no name at the time except "The Rife machine." BSRR is just my term for it. I think that this name is an appropriate description of the technology. There is a big overlap in the meanings of waves and radiation, so this can be a bit confusing. For a normal average individual to understand the technology, we will have to have a quick look into the basics of quantum mechanics and nature of the universe or nature of the matter. Quantum mechanics is fundamental to explaining the functioning of systems at atomic length scales and smaller and is in the base of physics and define the way that we comprehend the world scientifically. One of the most important experiments in quantum mechanics and in science that defined the way we perceive the world is experiment known as the double slit experiment. It is also the experiment that did not just define our world but also created the biggest problem in science so far that is still "in the air" and nobody especially scientists do not like to talk about it and avoid the subject. If we have a barrier like a wall with two slits in it. Imagine throwing balls at the wall. Some will bounce off, but some will hit the slits. If there's another wall behind the first, the balls that have gone through the slits will hit it. If you identify all the points where a ball has hit the other wall, what do you expect to see? Two strips of marks approximately the identical appearance as the slits. So any time when you throw something that was made of atoms through the slits you will get the two strips of marks roughly the same shape as the slits. So far so good. But what if we shine a light (of a single color, that is, of a single wavelength) at a wall with two slits, or not just the light but any other form of a wave into it and not solid matter like electrons or atoms. What would we expect to see at the wall? As the wave passes through both slits

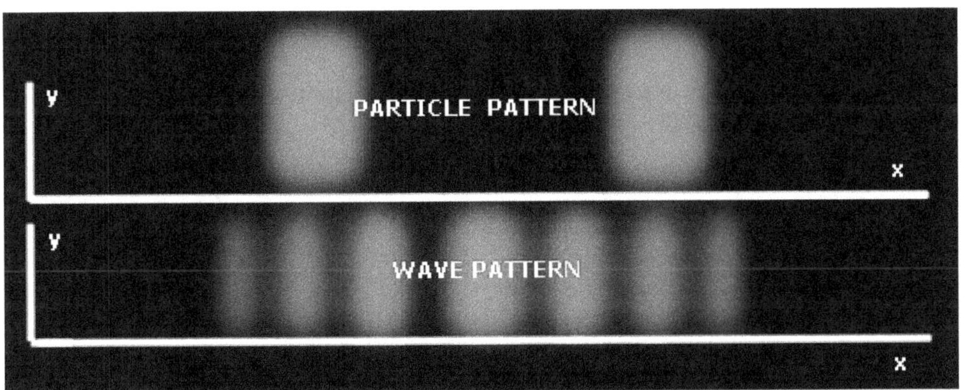

it basically divides into two new waves, each expanding out from one of the slits. The waves will interfere with each other. At some points, they will cancel each other out, and at others, where peak meets peak, they will reinforce each other and produce the strongest light. When the light goes through the slits you will see a stripe pattern on the second wall, many of the bright stripes called an interference pattern. So when we shot solid matter, we get two stripes when we shot wave we get the interference pattern. So far so good. Now what will happen if we instead of tennis balls shot solid matter from quantum realm like electrons through? They are matter like any other so we should expect just two strips. Actually, that is what is going to happen if we have just one slit. We will see that some of the particles will move through the open slit and hit the second wall. It was the same as the tennis balls would. The spots they arrive at form a strip roughly the same shape as the slit. But when we open the second slit, something unnatural happens. We would assume two rectangular strips on the second wall, as with the tennis balls, but what you see is very different. The spots where electrons hit build up to replicate the interference pattern from a wave. So again when we open the second slit we have unnatural interference pattern from a wave. How can this be? Because scientist could not explain this they theorized that somehow the electrons interfere with each other, so they do not arrive in the same places they would if they were alone. To counter that they did the experiment by shooting individual electrons one at the time. However, the interference pattern continues still if you shoot the electrons one by one. So there is something seriously wrong here. Electrons had no interfering. Strangely, each individual electron contributes one dot to an overall pattern that looks like the interference pattern of a wave. So again how could that be?

We perceive the world in solid form. We think that matter exist and that the universe is solid. We define our reality by the solidity of the matter. How could we live in the reality that is not solid but just made out of the waves? It is not possible. It would mean everything we perceive is just an illusion and that in reality matter is just a wave that we perceive as a solid matter. It is not possible and we need explanation or we need to redefine religion. Could it be that each electron somehow splits, passes through both slits at once, interferes with itself, and then recombines to meet the second screen as a single, localized particle? To figure this out, we can install a detector by the splits, to detect which slit an electron moves through. And that is when the seriousness comes in. Like it is already not enough that matter equally doesn't exist and that everything is just the wave but wait there is more. The nightmare of the scientific community. If you do that, place a detector by the slits, then the pattern on the detector screen turns into the particle pattern of two strips! The interference pattern vanishes. Somehow, the act of watching makes sure that the electrons travel like well-behaved little tennis balls. They knew they were being observed and then form the pattern of the regular solid matter. The act of observing by some form of intelligence forces the electrons (or any other form of mater) into its solid form. Conclusion of this scientific experiment was that all the matter is actually the wave and let say "download" itself into the solid matter only when observed by intelligence. So any matter has duality in itself. It is the famous wave-particle duality of quantum mechanics that defines our way of scientific looking at the universe. This phenomenon has been confirmed for elementary particles, but also for compound particles like atoms and even molecules. So basically everything around us is just a wave. Niels Bohr viewed the "duality paradox" as an essential or metaphysical fact of nature. As Albert Einstein wrote: "It seems as though we must use sometimes the one theory and sometimes the other, while at times we may use either. We are faced with a new kind of difficulty. We have two contradictory pictures of reality; separately neither of them fully explains the phenomena of light, but together they do."

However, scientists do not tell it all. They do not like this experiment too much because even today it is a big "mystery" of quantum mechanics. A scientist will say when asked that it is just measurement problem of quantum mechanics. However, it is not. They are scared of it. They do not have the explanation that can go along with an acceptable way of looking at things, so they ignore the experiment. For example, the scientist at Washington University found that: "Quasi-measurements cause the zeno effect, possibly explaining why the particles do not form an interference pattern if one detects which slit they pass through." Somehow they seem to be leaving out the fact that the difference occurs only when particles are being actively observed. Scientists may ignore the findings, but they still accept the result of experiment and will define it as what they call the dualistic nature of matter. What we accept as particles, such as electrons, or atoms, or molecules, somehow combine characteristics of particles and characteristics of waves. That is the famous wave-particle duality of quantum mechanics.

So if the matter is just a wave, then it would have all the characteristic of the wave. The height of a wave, is called its amplitude, distance from a particular point on one wave, to the same point on the next is called the wavelength and most importantly the number of waves passing every second is called frequency, f. Frequency is ranked in units called hertz (Hz). The faster a wave is traveling, the higher its frequency but, the shorter its wavelength. When waves of the same frequency come into contact, they are going to combine into one wave with larger amplitude, or greater energy if you like. It is called resonance. A well-known model is a playground swing, which works like a pendulum. Pushing a child in a swing in time with the natural interval of the swing (its resonant frequency) produces the swing to go higher and higher (maximum amplitude).

This is because the energy the swing absorbs is maximized when the pushes match the swing's natural oscillations. So if the matter is just the wave then what defines different matter. Well as it turns out, the lower the frequency the density of the matter is stronger. And every particle, atom or molecule has its own frequency in which it can resonate. Different atoms different frequency for all of the matter in the universe.

There is a good quote from Nikola Tesla who said: "If you want to find the secrets of the universe, think in terms of energy, frequency, and vibration." If a frequency of one wave is extremely different then a frequency of another wave they will not just resonate, but they will not ever interact with each other at all. The two can occupy the same time and space. A good example of this are the waves that go into your cell phone. You can go inside the solid building but you will still have the signal on your phone, and the waves will go through the walls literally. However, if you have resonance, you can combine the energies to make some "destruction." Balanced twisting that produced in the 1940 failure of Galloping Gertie, the original Tacoma Narrows Bridge, is characterized as an example of a resonance phenomenon. Armies have to break the step when crossing over the bridges. Alternatively, you can scream at wine glass to shatter it. Voice can hit resonance of glass at 550 Hz. It is in the human voice range. Such a strong, solid form like glass can shatter just from the sound. Everything has a frequency, even planet Earth itself. It is known as the Schumann resonance. What do you believe will occur if someone decided to bombard the Earth with waves at a frequency of Schumann resonance? There will be resonance with earth and if enough energy is sent that energy will not be able to dissipate naturally in time but will start to accumulate and at the end will release itself in the form of an artificially created earthquake.

First, artificially created earthquake was created back in 1898 by Tesla. Besides all of the credited work and all of the work that other "great scientist" stole from him he was also credited to have worked on unknown energy-sources, to be contacted by UFOs, caused the Tunguska explosion by a death-ray, and even worked on an earthquake-generator. Tesla said the oscillator was around 7 inches (18 cm) long, and weight one or two pounds; something: "You could put in your overcoat pocket." At one point while experimenting with the oscillator, he alleged it generated a resonance in several buildings causing complaints to the police. What happened was that he placed his tiny vibrator in his coat-pocket and went out to seek a half-erected steel building. He found one in the Wall Street district. It was just steel and didn't have the brick. He assembled the device to one of the beams. Tesla said that eventually the structure began to creak and weave and the steel-workers came to the ground panic-stricken, believing that there had been an earthquake. Police and ambulance were called. Ten minutes more and he would have laid the building to the street with something that you can put in your pocket. That is the power of resonance. However, his "telegeodynamics" system never managed to get beyond the prototype, but he also imagined using the oscillations generated by his device to prospect the underground. It is basic idea that all modern seismologists also use.

Today we use resonance in medicine too. For example, the hydrogen atoms in water are just protons. The protons have a resonant frequency that they vibrate (inside the huge magnetic field of an MRI machine). And that resonant frequency is in the radio range. When you are in the MRI machine, radio waves are hitting the water in your body, making the protons (hydrogen atoms) to vibrate (resonate) at that same frequency. Vibrating protons give off their own radio signal, and that signal is used to build a picture of your watery leg/brain/belly. It is magnetic. It is resonance. It is imaging. MRI. Alternatively, you can bombard the water with its own water molecule frequency instead of the frequency of the protons. That will destroy the bond and force hydrogen and oxygen to split out of H2O. It is electrolysis just hundreds of times more efficient than regular one. It is allegedly so efficient that there are even some patents and claims that you can run your car on that alone. You ever heard of a water power car? Probably not but it was called Dune Buggy by its inventor Stan Meyers. He experimented with resonance in his garage and used BSRR instead of regular electrolysis to break the water molecules. Pentagon showed lots of interest in that project. They even sent some of their men to look into it. He drove his Dune Buggy for a news report on Ohio TV station and also calculated that from Los Angeles to New York it will use 22 gallons of water. Supposedly. There is no documented evidence that the system provides sufficient hydrogen to run an engine. Philip Ball, writing in academic journal Nature, characterized Meyer's claims as pseudoscience, noting that: "It's not easy to establish how Meyer's car was meant to work, except that it involved a fuel cell that was able to split water using less energy than was released by recombination of the elements ...". But what was not the pseudoscience, was the money. He was offered a bribe for patent and for him to go away from rich investors in the amount of no less than 1 billion dollars. Billion with the B. He refused. He wanted to put his invention into commercial use and was Christian and didn't like "One World Government" and wanted to give people self-sufficiency. Stanley Meyer departed suddenly on March 21, 1998, after eating at a restaurant. Conspiracy theorists insist that he was killed to suppress the technology and that the United States government were involved in his death.

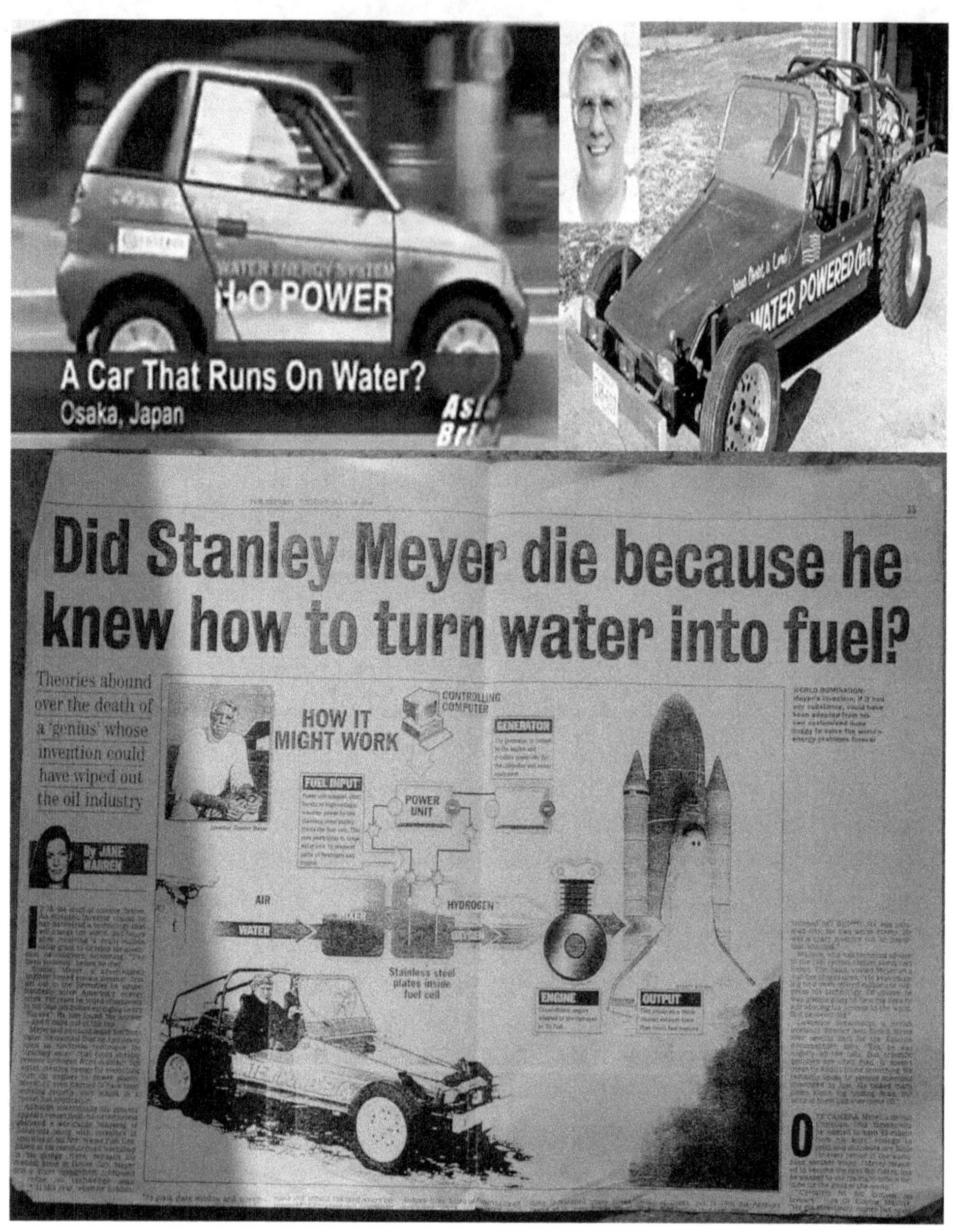

His brother claimed that during a meeting with two Belgian investors in a restaurant: "Stanley took a sip of cranberry juice. Then he grabbed his neck, bolted out the door, dropped to his knees and vomited violently. I ran outside and asked him, 'What's wrong?'". He said: "They poisoned me", and died. Mayer water fuel cell was later examined by three expert witnesses in court who found there was nothing revolutionary about the cell at all and it was simply using conventional electrolysis. However, it is possible that they did not understand the technology behind double slit experiment. To date, no one reproduced his technology commercially or at least that I know of. There is just couple more cases of individual inventors who made water cars with a similar approach like Herman P. Anderson who actually used little bit different approach and deuterium (heavy water) was essential to his fuel cell. Herman was consulted with Nasa and the US Airforce on some of country's most important Top Secret Projects including the first US satellite in space, the SR-71 Blackbird, the Stealth Fighter/Bomber and Star Wars. Herman worked closely with Nazi operation paperclip refugee Dr. Wernher von Braun testing hydrogen-powered rocket engines, and he also worked with engineers at the now famous Skunk Works, the Jet Propulsion Laboratory, JPL, and Cal Tech. The government of the State of Tennessee allowed him to drive his water powered car but had forbidden him to try to use his invention commercially. In any normal free country, he would be glorified as the man who freed the world from poverty. And yes most of our modern economy depends on energy consumption. With free energy, there would be no poverty and no environmental destruction, but there would also be an uncontrollable, independent, self-sufficient population with no interest in war or obedience to corporate overloads and government. Imagine a world where energy is free and safe and out of governmental control. There is one more case in Japan. They produced a water powered car in 2008 that only runs on air and water. You can see it on the picture. It is not salt water battery electric car that is available commercially today, but again one more real water powered car. Not surprisingly, there has been little to no coverage of this car in America or anywhere else. There was another good quote from Tesla life when he was confronted by J.P Morgan for his free wireless electric energy tower experiments. He said to him: "Ok, where exactly am I going to put my ampere meter? "

However, what about the medicine. Does cancer have resonance? Alternatively, haw about HIV? Royal Raymond Rife developed technology which is still commonly used today in the fields of optics, microscopy, electronics, radiochemistry, biochemistry, ballistics, and aviation and particularly in imaging and medical microscopy. In life, he was awarded 14 different rewards. Rife attended Heidelberg University in Germany. He received there honorary Doctor of Parasitology degree. Rife also in 1936 received an honorary Doctor of Science degree from the University of Southern California. Rifle's inventions include the heterodyning ultraviolet microscope, a micro dissector, and a micromanipulator. He was not just some quack like most of the "educated" people in the field of medicine will like you to believe. His original business while still attending the university was with the firm of Carl Zeiss, at their New York City offices and later at their offices in Germany where he worked directly with Carl Zeiss, Hans Luckel and other scientists in the research, design, and production of excellent microscopes. He spent five years working with that group while he was attending the University of Heidelberg. It is stated that Rife worked with the United States Navy before and during World War One and that he was commissioned as a Lt. Commander USNR. During the years just before the great depression, Dr. Rife worked for both the United States Government and the Carl Zeiss Optics firm. At one period, his monetary base dissolved and he took a job as a chauffeur for multimillionaire Henry Timkin. Dr. Rife's association with Henry Timkin served well for both of them. Timkin fabricated roller bearings. Some of the bearings were crumbling down due to imperfections in the steel used to create the bearings. Rife designed and built an X-ray device that monitored every bearing getting out and discarded every faulty one before it could be sent out as a finished product. He saved the company millions. Timkin was so satisfied that he established a monthly lifetime payment to Rife for providing the specialized X-ray machine for his production environment. Henry Timkin and his partner, Bridges remained so fascinated with Dr. Rife and his work that they set up a fund to finance a wholly equipped laboratory at Point Loma, California and to carry the expenses of a research program in the laboratory that was created. In the laboratory mentioned above, he performed most of his experiments. At one point, Rife had as many as twelve laboratory assistants working for him. In 1916 most powerful microscopes could reach a magnification of 2500 diameters. With this instrument, a scientist could see parasites, mold and many bacteria, but no one had seen a virus. Rife built a magnifying instrument that worked on a different principle than the existing microscopes of his day. The first microscope that enabled him to see a virus was built in 1920. Rife was the creator of the Universal Microscope which he introduced to the world in 1933 as the world most powerful microscope. One of the various attractive characteristics of this microscope is that, in contrast to the Electron Microscope, the Universal Microscope does not kill the specimens under observation and allows observation of actual living specimens in all conditions, indicating it does not rely on fixing or staining to render visibility or definition. With his microscope, Rife became the first human being actually to see a live virus, and until quite recently, the Universal Microscope was the only one who was able to observe living viruses. Modern electron microscopes instantly kill everything. The rife microscope can see the bustling activity of living viruses as they change form to accommodate changes in an environment, replicate rapidly in response to carcinogens, and transform normal cells into tumor cells. Rife managed this by utilizing various forms of lighting to bring the virus within visibility. He first used the technique of using light to stain the subjects because he understood that the particles of the chemical stains were much too large to enter into the structures he attempted to visualize.

Furthermore, stains used in microscopy are often lethal to the specimens. One factor allowing these original images was Rife's use of a tool called a Risley counter-rotating prism. The refracted and polarized ray will turn normally hidden organism that is invisible into becoming visible in color particular to their structure or chemical make-up. All optical elements were made of block quartz, which permits the passage of ultraviolet rays. By this means Rife had found out that different bacteria and viruses glow at different frequencies. This proved that organisms could be classified by their index of refraction or in another word their resonance frequency. In other words, he found out that they vibrate under different frequencies. Rife slowly classified the unique spectroscopic signature of each microbe, using a slit spectroscope attachment. Then, he gradually twisted prisms to focus light of an individual wavelength upon the microorganism he was examining. Then it resonated with the spectroscopic signature frequency of the microbe based on the now-established fact that every molecule oscillates at its distinct frequency.

Utilizing a resonant wavelength micro-organism that cannot be seen in white light suddenly become visible as a flash of light when they are exposed to the color frequency that resonates with their distinct spectroscopic signature. Rife was capable of seeing those otherwise invisible organisms and watch them how they behave. He could view organisms that no one else could see with ordinary microscopes.

Rife was so far ahead of his co-workers in the 1930s that it was hard for them to understand what he was actually doing without traveling directly to San Diego to Rife's laboratory to look for themselves through his Virus Microscope. And several did precisely that. One was Virginia Livingston. She ultimately went from New Jersey to Rife's Point Loma (San Diego) neighborhood to live and became a regular visitor to his lab. Virginia Livingston is now given credit for identifying the organism which causes human cancer, based on research papers she published in 1948. The real truth is that Rife had identified the human cancer virus in 1920. He called the cancer virus 'Cryptocides primordiales.' Virginia Livingston renamed it to 'Progenitor Cryptocides.' Royal Rife was never even stated in her papers. In fact, Rife rarely got credit for his monumental discoveries. He was a modest, humble scientist, committed to expanding his discoveries rather than to ambition, fame, and glory. He started research work on tuberculosis in 1920. In a short time, it became clear to Rife there was more involved in this disease then bacterium. This encouraged him to develop virus microscopes, of which two preceded the Universal. Rife was the first scientist to isolate and photographed active tuberculosis as well as many other viruses. Rife also worked in isolating a virus specific to cancer, seeing it gave off a unique purple-red emanation. There was no success until Rife by mistake left a tube in the light of an ionizing lamp. He noticed the tube became clouded, registering activity. His work led to the first successful culturing of the virus outside a living host in history. Rife extracted the cancer virus from a human breast mass. He filtered, cultured and re-cultured these over ten times over a two hundred and forty-hour period. They inserted the last generation culture into the live rat. The rat would inevitably develop cancer. Rife would then extract cancer, extract the virus, and repeat the process. He did this procedure over four hundred times.

After Dr. Rife discovered how to see a virus, the next logical step became to devise a method to kill the virus or microbe without damage to the host. Since the days of Nikola Tesla and his work, men of science had known of the connection of frequencies with the operation of the human body and the matter in general. So Rife turned to electromagnetic frequencies because he could detect the bacteria and virus unique frequencies with his microscope and then expose them and watch the effects. He found that each microorganism had a distinct frequency to which it resonates to and was defenseless. Rife termed this the "mortal oscillatory rate." Over and over again he would observe the virus absorbing energy until it dies when a certain frequency was applied. Sometimes they even exploded. He created charts revealing which frequency settings would kill which microbe or virus. If he had not invented his microscope, there would have been no treatment based on resonance. Numerous reports and news stories emerged concerning these extraordinary achievements. His work became known to many of the physicians in the Southern California area. Some of them even came from all over the United States to observe what he was doing and verify his results. During November 1931, Dr. Milbank Johnson called forty-four Los Angeles area doctors to his home in Pasadena, California to acknowledge Rife

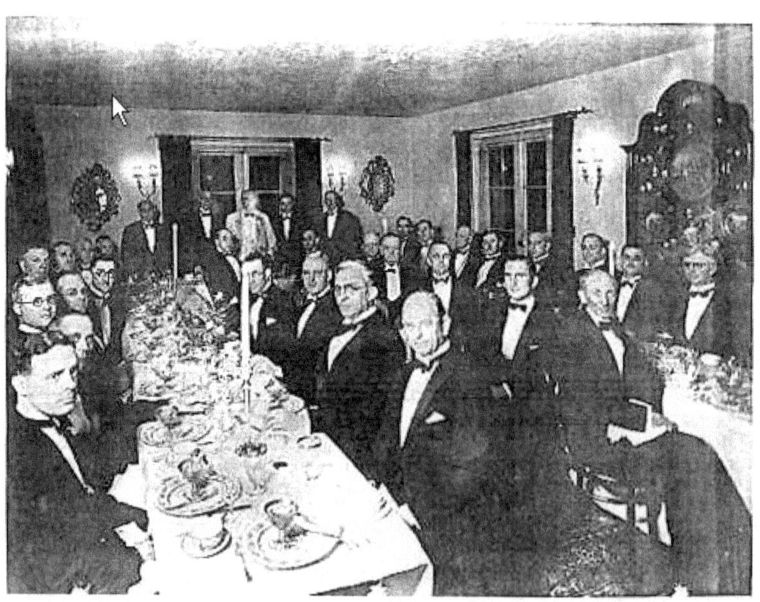

On November 20, 1931, forty-four of the nation's most respected medical authorities honored Royal Rife with a banquet billed as "The End To All Diseases" at the Pasadena estate of Dr Milbank Johnson.

for the work he was performing. Dr. Royal Rife was acknowledged as the man who ended all disease that ever existed. Well, at least the ones that are infectious and can be bombarded with resonance. The banquet was even called "The End of All Disease."

It was the first time in history when terminally ill cancer patient was healed completely. Fourteen of the patients became completely free of any cancer at that time. The therapy was then adjusted, meaning the resonant frequency and the remaining two patients also responded. The recovery rate for patients that have non-treatable cancer and was declared terminally ill by accepted medical industry with using Rife's technology was 100%. Through 1939 Dr. Rife was formally summoned to address the Royal Society of Medicine in London, England, which had verified his findings. He was further received invitations to lecture in France and Germany. Dr. R. Seidel described and formally published the Rife Ray Tube system therapy for the treatment of cancer in the journal of the Franklin Institute during February 1944. Dr. Rife's treatments of the virus and bacterial infections and his microscopes were described and praised by the Smithsonian Institute in an article published in the Institute's publication during 1944. A report from the Smithsonian Institution confirms Rife's work. Titled "The New Microscope" by Dr. R.E. Seidel (report #3781) it states: "Under the Universal Microscope disease organisms such as those of cancer ... and another disease may be observed to succumb when exposed to certain lethal frequencies..."

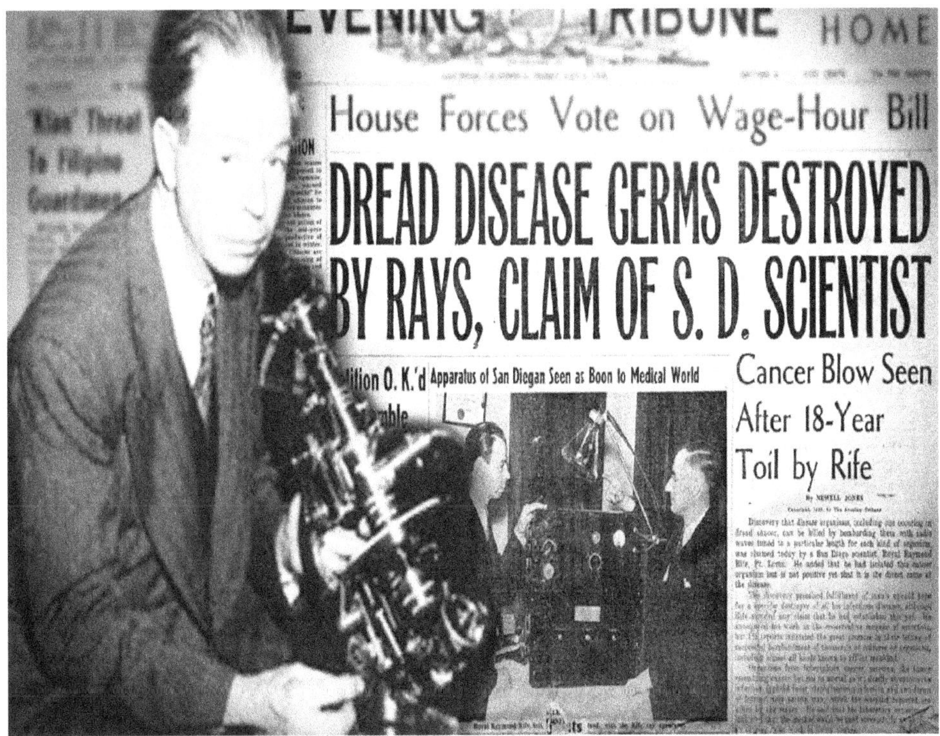

It took a Rife long time, years of his life, working 48 hours at a time until he detected the frequencies which explicitly destroyed herpes, polio, spinal meningitis, tetanus, influenza, and an immense number of other dangerous disease organisms.

At first, an attempt was made to buy out Rife. Morris Fishbein, a physician who became the editor of the Journal of the American Medical Association, sent an attorney to Rife with "an offer he can't refuse." Rife refused. We will never know the exact terms of this offer but it is highly likely they did not want for his machine to become commercially available. They probably tried to bribe him to destroy his invention. For example, when Fishbein made a similar offer to Hoxsey, and he declined. Fishbein used his immensely strong governmental associations to have Hoxsey arrested 125 times in 16 months. The charges were always thrown out of court, but the harassment continued. It became so bad that AMA posted flyers in every post office in the entire country for scaring people of using Hoxsey and any other alternative cancer treatments. However, what we need to understand is that he did not act alone. He was just AMA front man at the time. Later in 1961, he became the founding Editor of Medical World News, a magazine for doctors. In 1970 he endowed the Morris Fishbein Center for the study of the history of science and medicine at the University of Chicago.

However, Fishbein and the AMA must have recognized that this approach would backfire if used on Rife. They could not arrest Rife as they could Hoxsey for practicing medicine without the license. Also, the trial that was compiled on trumped-up charges would mean that prominent medical authorities working with Rife would introduce their testimony supporting Rife and the word of his invention would come out to the general public. The defense would surely introduce evidence such as the 1934 medical study done with USC. If they have a public trial about a painless therapy that cured 100% of the terminal cancer patients with medical proof and also the cost is nothing but a little electricity. Well, that was not what powers at be wanted. Rife didn't just dropped from nowhere. He was a well-known scientist that had spent decades collecting precise evidence of his work. He had film and stop-motion photographs that could be released to the public and so on. Killing him directly will just made things worse.

They had to use different tactics and they were utilized. The first incident was the gradual disappearing of film, photographs, components, written records and other evidence from Rife's lab. The culprit was never caught. Then, while Rife tried to replicate his missing data (when computers were not available), someone vandalized his expensive virus microscopes. Then entire laboratory "mysteriously" burned at the time when the men running the laboratory was visiting Rife in San Diego. Then papers in Rife's laboratory in San Diego "mysteriously" disappeared, as did parts of his microscopes. Final blow happened later when police illegally seized the rest of Rife's 50 years of research. The physician who helped the most Dr. Royal Rife to receive recognition for his work was Dr. Milbank Johnson. One day he was taken to the hospital for what was thought to be a minor problem by attending physicians during 1944 but he "mysteriously" died there of food poisoning. Rife and partners had set up a company called the Ray Beam Tube Corporation to build the Rife Machine. He had given employment and a contract to an engineer to handle production. Fishbein supposedly supported the engineer to bring suit against Rife. A suit was long and expensive. Rife won, but the cost of the suit caused the financial destruction of the company and in time of great depression end of production. A huge pile of cash was spent to ensure that doctors who had seen Rife's therapy and knew about his work would forget everything or else were threatened by the American Medical Association and the State of California with the loss of their licenses if they continued on the program. Arthur Kendall, who worked with Rife on the cancer virus, accepted almost a quarter of a million dollars to suddenly retire in Mexico. Dr. George Dock, who collaborated with Rife, was silenced with an enormous grant, along with the highest honors the AMA could bestow. Dr. Couche also gave up Rife's work and went back to prescribing drugs.

This battle emotionally destroyed Rife himself and his entire program dissolved. Loss of his lab and mental and emotional results of the lawsuit was enough to make Rife to became an alcoholic. During 1950 Rife worked to improve energy instruments with John Crane. John Crane ended up with the right to the microscopes. During 1960 Medical officials invaded Crane's lab and confiscated all of the devices and records. That was not enough, so he was also charged by the State of California for committing the fraud and sent to prison. Rife is said to have escaped to Mexico at this time. He did not work with no one after that last incident. Rife died in 1971, at Grossman Hospital in El Cajon, California of a heart attack after spending the last years of his life in an El Cajon nursing home. He was without friends or funds. He discovered an incredibly simple, electronic approach to curing all diseases. He made the low-cost discovery that could end the suffering of countless millions. It would have changed the life on Earth forever. Surely, the medical world would rush to embrace it with every imaginable accolade and financial reward imaginable. You have contracted a universal cure which makes drugs obsolete, and the only cost of using it is electricity so the pharmaceutical industry might be thrilled to hear about your work. Of course, some of you may regard this as just an amusing piece of fiction. Do your own research and believe whatever you want. In reality, this technology could have a great potential if properly developed. The only question here is could you target all of the viruses or just some of them. We know he cured cancer in 100 percent range. However, if the resonance of microbes is too close to the rest of the human cells radiation would transfer some of the energy to them burning regular tissue, but if the frequency is distinctive, then this might work. Today, for example, there are thousands of people who have a Lyme Disease diagnosis, but antibiotic treatment is not producing long-term relief. Rife machine therapy is turning out to be valuable and only available long-term therapy in existence for Lyme Disease. But we would never really know. The magnitude of this insane crime eclipses every mass murder in history.

Now let us look into the food industry. We might think that there is nothing there and that food industry is just regular business, but the situation is much more complicated than that. The food industry is controlled by the same group of people that control big pharmaceutical companies and that control all other international companies by big extent. It is the same oligarchy over and over again. Food is something very existential, and it is something very fundamental to human existence from the beginning of time. Even if we do not understand what is going on, people are going to be naturally suspicious if they suspect that their food is chemically enriched or genetically modified. They are going to ask questions that don't directly concern them such as: Why there is hunger in the world? Secrecy of corporations is just going to heighten the suspicion. Even if you do not understand what is going on you will see that small farmers around the world are in trouble and that every year they are being pushed out of business by some number. And why are they in trouble? Well, there is too much food in the world, and it suppresses the prices. Not the prices in supermarkets that you pay, just the wholesale prices in which farmers are selling to big food companies for further distribution that are highly susceptible to crop, seeds or products that will reduce their costs even if the long term effect is detrimental to the soil and environment. You can see this in India, America, you see it in Canada, Argentina. It is the strategy to undermine small farmer's livelihoods.

Five agro-chemical corporations control around 85% of the entire world food markets and what they want to do is to gain control over the entire food chain, from the seeds to the table. Hunger is not a technological problem. The world produces enough food. There are hungry people because the food is not distributed to them. It is a problem of concentration of food production and trade in the hands of an agro-chemical cartel that does not want to give access to undeveloped countries as a tool of social and political control and especially the population control. It is not a money issue but the issue that is more in the line of eugenic protocols for depopulation. The cause of food deficit was not natural but was a result of the western financial policy. Considering the global population is now at 7.2 billion, in the lack of population control in their mind and some Pentagon projections, these 7.2 billion would become 14 billion by 2040, 28 billion by 2070 and 56 billion by the end of the 21st century. This is clearly in their mind an unsustainable growth given that we live on a finite planet, and that we now use almost 40% of the earth's ice-free landmass to feed ourselves. There are no more landmasses to discover and exploit, we have destroyed the planet's life maintenance systems and have polluted the soil and the sea. "It is questionable," Kissinger once gloated: "Whether aid donor countries will be prepared to provide the sort of massive food aid called for by the import projections on a continuing long-term basis. The large-scale famine of a kind not experienced for several decades a kind the world thought had been permanently banished was foreseeable famine." This "return of famines" would not be possible without the participation of multinational corporations. It is politics that create the difference in times of famine. Food stocks are not significantly decreased as we might be thinking. Food is sold on the food market to those that can afford the higher prices. That is not the poor and rural populations of Africa, and this is done deliberately. Uneven distribution of food is a geopolitical decision, and that is the problem rather than the ratio of food to people. Also, wars and the shifts of an industry that can create a vulnerable imbalance in nation's economies are important constituents. In developing nations, when population quits farming to work in industry and technologies, food prices are going to rise. A developing country with people struggling to raise its living standards would buy the cheapest food, and that is what agro companies are glad to provide.

A political strategy used in collaboration with international food cartels is to undermine a third world nations farming production creating dependence on imports. As small farms disappear, withholding food or raising prices can then be strategically used as a war strategy to coerce cooperation. The countries resources are siphoned elsewhere through importing food that could be supplied from within. Control of an entire economy and the nation that relies on imports of food is easily accomplished. Not with war, but with food, or the lack of it. However, if it is a war that is wanted for a regime change, a hungry, rioting population certainly delivers. Poverty and social collapse are the goals behind the last 50 years of the globalization of agriculture. British neo-imperial plans upon nation-states. Policies which destroy the primary requirement for national survival: food self-sufficiency. In the US self-sufficiency for expanding population was created with the industrialization of agriculture and the invention of agribusiness. With industrialized farming production of food had a lower and lower cost. In time small farmer disappeared and was replaced with food cartels. Now, the portion of the US population that is self-sufficient and are producing their own food is 2-3%, a shift from 1870 when it was between 70-80%. Also the population is much larger then in 1870. If something like great depression strikes again, there would be no food for the vast amount of population that would depend on the government for survival. Food shortages seem remote and unreal in this land of plenty.

For "safety" reasons a heavily protested bill, S 510, The Food Safety Modernization Act was passed, and intent is the same as in policies forced upon the developing nations. To bury the small farmer. Additional concern over the bill is that the language allows for regulation over homegrown foods as well. The Food Safety Modernization Act looks like it is headed to become law. It is being hailed as a breakthrough achievement in food safety, and it would hand vast new powers and funding to the FDA so that it can clean up the food supply and "protect" all Americans from food-borne pathogens. There's just one problem with all this. It is all a big lie. Moreover, even without the imposition of food supervision laws, the patenting of engineered seeds as a product has shifted the whole idea of food rights, utilizing what was once very simple into a complex problem. GMO seeds can be engineered to commit suicide after one harvest, leaving the farmer dependent on the corporation providing the seed. Farmers must also use the chemical herbicides and pesticides that these seeds are engineered to tolerate. Through the inevitability of cross-contamination, these genetically modified, patented organisms could invade the entire food supply. Pollen flies to non-GMO crops and pollinates them making half GMO hybrids. The effort by these corporations has gone so far ahead that they have set a precedent by successfully suing farmers whose crops have been cross-contaminated with patented genetic material. The wind blows pollen on your normal corn, and then you are going to court. And that reveals the intent.

A number of African countries suffering from the worst food shortages have learned the lesson and will not allow GMO seeds into their countries, even in the form of food aid, without it being first milled to prevent it from being planted. To survive into the future because of all of the overpopulation issue, the oligarchy is now "forced" to erect a global governing structure authorized to wield global governing instruments capable of maintaining "peace" among men, of establishing harmony between man and nature, and of forging continuity between this and future generations. They must, in other words, consider not only what is good for us here and now but what is good for future generations and all life on Earth and they must respond accordingly. Population control is the most urgent step needed of us here and now if we are to preserve our existence. Therefore, population control must and will be declared a Planetary Security Prerogative. Standard is a report by ten British writers, some of them from the U.K. Office of Science that represent government official policy, in Science magazine, "Food Security: The Challenge of Feeding 9 Billion People" (February 12, 2010). They conclude: "Any optimism must be tempered by the enormous challenges of making food production sustainable while controlling greenhouse gas emission and conserving dwindling water supplies, as well as meeting the Millennium Development Goal of ending hunger..." Necessary on feeding "9 billion people by 2050" has grown the be sick line expression for demanding still more globalization and more control. The crude estimation is that for today's 7.2 billion people, around 4 billion tons of annual grain production is the level needed for adequate diets, in the form of personal cereals consumption and for feeding the farm animals, and for reserves. The underproduction of grains had a worsening additive effect. And by the way all of this is just justification behind real policies of crypto eugenics made to be stealthy and pushed into the UN as a form of warfare.

Because of demand for oil, world's grain and oilseed crops are going into biofuels. In the US, which alone produces around 40% of world corn (maize) production, 40% of the entire corn crop went for fuel, ethanol. The International Institute for Sustainable Development estimates that the CO2 and climate benefits from replacing petroleum fuels with biofuels like ethanol are zero. Protecting the environment is a lie. It is again policy of crypto eugenics. Biofuels do have direct, emissions that are typically 30–90% lower than those for gasoline or diesel fuels. However, since for some biofuels, indirect emissions that include land use change, water scarcity, loss of biodiversity and nitrogen pollution through the excessive use of fertilizers can led to greater total emissions than when using petroleum products. Around 60 nations having biofuel mandates. The debate between ethanol and food has become a moral issue. In 2007, the global cost of corn doubled as a consequence of an outburst in ethanol production in the US. Because corn is the cheapest as animal feed the price of dairy products, meat, eggs, and cereals rose as well. World grain reserves decreased to less than two months, the lowest level in over 30 years. Further unintended results from the rise in ethanol production incorporate the significant rise in land rents, the rise in natural gas and chemicals used for fertilizers, over-pumping of aquifers like the Ogallala, cutting even more forests to plant plants for fuel, return of harmful methods as edge tillage. Edge tillage is the practice of planting all the way to the edge of the field. This is bad because it removes protecting bordering plants and that results in chemical runoff from the field and soil erosion. It took 40 years to end edge tillage in the US.

Brazil relied massively on imported oil and therefore was under political pressure from oil controlling forces. For self-sufficiency, they decided to plant crops for the production of biofuels. In their tropical climate, that can give high yields of sugar cane. The government developed the most extensive fuel ethanol program in the world in the 1990s. They genetically modified fermenting bacteria to withstand high alcohol concentration and now are entirely fuel independent based on domestic sugar cane and soybeans production. As a consequence, Brazil is cutting nearly a million acres of tropical forest per year to produce biofuel from these crops. The result is about 50% more carbon emitted by using these biofuels than using petroleum fuels. The political imposition of the system of biofuels is undermining the capacity of the US farm belt and agriculture everywhere. In the traditional US corn belt now, instead of high-tech farmers, industry, and regional food production (milk, orchards, diversified crops, meat animals), the pattern is a monoculture, imported food, and ghost towns. Enforcing these models is an interlock of cartels of mega-companies in fertilizers, agrochemicals, processing and distribution, integrated into policy with the WTO, World Bank, and IMF, and private, London-centered financial networks. Even more corporate dominance and a smaller number of small farmers dependent on international trade control by five companies.

The entire world grain trade is controlled by Cargill, ADM, Bunge, Dreyfus, and very few others protected by the global political establishment and their institutions. For example, one central tenet of the WTO can speak for himself: the decree that no nation has the right to seek food self-sufficiency, but instead, must operate on the definition of "food security" as "access to world markets." What this means is if you do not want economic sanctions to be imposed by US, EU and others you must obey. This was declaration introduced in the GATT Uruguay Round (1984-94). It is a stealth way to attack an individual and especially small developing countries and their national sovereignty. The establishing rules of the WTO justified its claim that member-nations have no right to support their own farmers because that would be "depriving their citizenry" of the right to access to superior world markets for potentially cheaper and better food. Controlled by a cartel of course. Behind this and other fallacies stand the same Anglo-imperial globalist banking and commodities cartels. The record of destruction is awful.

We can take Mexico as a good example. In the 1960s, Mexico was a net food exporter, with water-management projects planned, a program for nuclear power development, and a growing industrial base. Utilizing collaboration between the governments of Mexico and the new nation of India, always food short under British rule, India became grain self-sufficient as of 1974. All this was ruined, following the 1980s attack for an excuse as free trade, then the 1992 NAFTA (North American Free Trade Alliance), and finally the 1995 WTO. Mexico was required to remove corn and beans production and became import-dependent, all the while, serving as a cheap-labor outsourcing zone for cartel exports of frozen foods and fresh produce for the US market. Now, hunger stalks Mexico. Millions fled looking for work and drug-running and death are displacing the farming that remains. This is the successful result of the British free-trade agriculture program.

The definition of genocide is action to exterminate a group of people deliberately. That applies equally to those who devise and implement policies politically. British imperialists have forever favored the stealth method, wishing to let others get their hands dirty while they can play innocent pushing their agenda further. This has definitely been the case with food policy, created for population control. Because of this policy, humankind has already reached the point where it is producing less than is required for its survival with the rising population in developing countries at the edge of hunger by design.

It all started a long time ago. Food was used as a weapon at least four millennia ago in Babylon. It all started after the Neolithic Revolution. The first excess of production was what created the first need for trade. So if you are stone age farmer and you produce more grain, then you can eat you would probably go down the hill to the fisherman village to trade some of your grains for fish. Then the population expanded and first city-states are formed. Then the first empires and so on. Eventually, the land was owned by lords and rest of the peasants were just slaves. In the time of Persia before Rome, there was already slavery and global scale food trading. From China and India to the Mediterranean. Then with the help of Phoenician fleet all over the Mediterranean and the Black Sea area. Already in antiquity the trade was booming. When Rome defeated Phoenicians in the Punic wars, it took over the trade. Actually to understand the economy of Rome is to understand the economy of the Persia because Romans as a tribe are from the Middle East not from Europe. They migrated to Europe from Asia Minor by colonization and by first eradicating by genocide real European people that lived in Apennine Peninsula known as Etruscans. They have brought with them the same culture and system that were present in the great empires like Assyria and Persia with them, the economy of scale based on trade and exes in food production control by a small number of traders and senators and oligarchs and slavery. Then they eradicated in genocide all of the people (meaning women and children also) that lived in Cartage, took over the trade routes and then moved to dominate the rest of Europe with a system that existed in the Asia Minor and the great empires of old. Don't forget history. It would be hard to understand the current world. We only have what we remember. Subdued external territories in Gaul, Brittany, Spain, Sicily, Egypt, North Africa, and the Mediterranean littoral had to ship grain to the noble Roman families, as taxes and tribute. Usually, the grain tax was higher than the land could bear. The same Roman system was implemented in Feudal Europe after the collapse of the Western Roman Empire. The empire collapsed, but money in the coffers remained, and the people running the show just changed their names into something local or Christian and became traders, bankers, nobility or cardinals.

The city-state of Venice took over grain routes, particularly after the Fourth Crusade (1202-04). Crusade had one more important aspect except for religion. And that is regaining control back from the Islamists of the ancient Roman trade routes. The same oligarchy that had been running trade in the Roman Empire now ran Venice and its trade. The main Venetian thirteenth-century trading routes were eastern termini in Constantinople, the ports of the Oltremare (which were the lands of the crusading States), and Alexandria, Egypt. Products from these ports were shipped first to Venice, and then from there made their way up the Po Valley to markets in Lombardy, or over the Alpine passes to the Rhône and into France. Venetian trade extended to the India, China and Mongol empire in the East and France in the west.

Near the fifteenth century, Venice remained still very much a banking and merchant center. However, it had started to spread some of its grain and other trade to the ruling Burgundian duchy, whose current headquarters was Antwerp. This empire, including a big part of today France, continued from Amsterdam and Belgium to much of present-day Switzerland. Venetian-Lombard-Burgundian nexus, give birth to each of the food cartel's six leading grain companies. These companies were either founded or inherited a substantial part of its operations that they have today. By the eighteenth century, the British Levant and East India companies had absorbed many of these Venetian operations and extended the trade globally to the new colonies in the Americas and Africa to. However, it was just expansion by the same ruling elite. Oligarchy just moved its center of operation into the City of London (not the capital city of England and the United Kingdom, known as London, big difference) and expanded trade, banking and slavery to the global level.

In the nineteenth century, the City of London-based Baltic Mercantile and Shipping Exchange became the world's leading instrument for contracting for and shipping grain. And why did they move? In seventeen centuries there was a conflict between bankers and House of Stuart. Bankers of Europe had join forces and financed William of Orange who invaded England and disposed of Stuarts and became King William III of England. He was sovereign Prince of Orange from birth, Stadtholder of Holland, Zeeland, Utrecht, Gelderland and Overijssel in the Dutch Republic and with the help of bankers from 1672 King of England, Ireland, and Scotland. At the end of sixteen century England was financial ruin. Gold and silver reserves were spent, civil war has morphed into the war with France and Netherlands in the next 50 years. The land was in bad shape, and William could not pay the army. He needed the money, and he excepted the "help" from the bankers but with one small counter favor. They asked to open their private bank that will have the status of the central bank. In return, they will bring gold as deposits which will be the bases to print money that will be lent to the state. So that is how in 1694 the Bank of England was created, the first private central bank in the world that had the right to print money (eventually out of nothing) legally. England as a state started to take the loans that were registered as a national debt. Over the period of 300 years, the oligarchy from Venice has spread to control trade and banking to France, Germany, Netherlands and eventually England. And by controlling England also controlling their rising colonies as well. Moving to England the Venice trade and banking families have practically just kept the power and wealth that they made back in the Roman Republic and expended their influence on America, Africa and big parts of Asia. The administrative headquarters are changed, and that is today the City of London. The City of London is a state, not a city, that contains the historic center and the primary central business district (CBD) of London. Now if you miss it read it again. The City of London is a state in London the same way the Vatican is country in Rome. It is also a county of England, being an enclave surrounded by Greater London. It does not fall under the legal system of Great Brittan. The City of London is considered to be sui generis, which is Latin for "in a class by itself." That it is one of the oldest self-governing local states in the world, with roots going back as far as medieval times when it was set up as a commune. Its right to exist predates that of parliament and even the Magna Carta of 1215, which was the charter of rights between King John and the barons, makes special reference to its "ancient liberties" and how they extend to all freemen of the realm. The status has afforded the jurisdiction a Lord Mayor since the days of William the Conqueror. The City of London is a state within a state. The deep state of western civilization if you like. The controlling center. The City of London Corporation prefers to view itself as an autonomous jurisdiction that defends the rights of freemen. Freemen are those considered not to be the property of a feudal lord but who enjoy privileges such as the right to earn money and own land. This has meant that the freemen of the City have uniquely benefited from the right to trade as merchants or members of a guild or livery. They also control their own police force operated and paid for by the City of London's own coffers and tax system. The City of London is real British "Crown" not the House of Windsor. Actually, Windsor is just name of the castle their real last name is Saxe-Coburg and Gotha (German: Sachsen-Coburg und Gotha). They changed it to Windsor to be more in line with the local population as a marketing move. Before the First World War, it was the family of the sovereigns of the United Kingdom, Belgium, Portugal, Bulgaria and branches of the family still reign in Belgium, the United Kingdom, and the other Commonwealth realms.

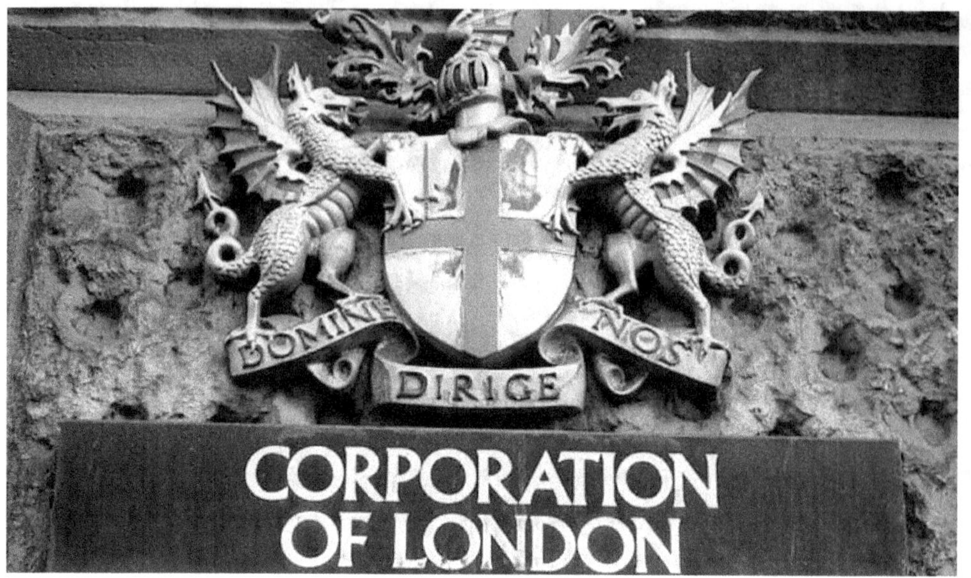

This trade structure to us mortals is mostly unknown. In the front of this trade structure in the City of London, is for the ceremonial and public eyes Mayor that they chose themselves without an election. They are just formally under House of Windsor but not in reality, and actually, I will correct myself, not even formally. Queen of England needs to ask for a permission from the Lord Mayor if she wants to visit the city. And she can do that only in the civil uniform. The Lord Mayor of London is the City of London's mayor and leader of the City of London Corporation. For instance, Sir Michael Bear and Sir Roger Gifford both were Lord Mayors of London. In both occasions, they welcomed the "Queen" in this manner. In full ceremonial uniform while the "Queen" was in civilian dress, standing one step below them.

For you, this might just be some coincidence or some irrelevant ceremonial show. It is because today you and most of the people in the schools have been learning that all of this is just history that has nothing to do with the modern world. It is just some reminisce of the past and that we today have democracy and human rights and laws and that there are UN and WTO beside governments just in case and other nice organizations that are there to help the world and to protect us from evil. The real reality is inverted, and your perception of reality is based on propaganda brainwashing emotional manipulation of social engineering schooling for masses. Freedom of information is freedom of choice. Wrong information, wrong perception, wrong choice with good intentions. Bank of England still stands with all of the influence and all of her creations like

Federal reserve of America and all other bank financed corporations, multinational companies, and businesses. Let us look just 100 years ago to see how had food business and trade had been organized. First company in the modern sense or one of the first was East India company. That is if we do not count The City of London Corporation. The Corporation's first recorded Royal Charter dates from around 1067 and actually had its privileges temporarily stripped by a writ quo warranto under Charles II in 1683, but they were later restored and confirmed by Act of Parliament under William III (one and the same "banking boy" of Orange) in 1690, after the "Glorious Revolution".

Power and control and economy and politics and war, it is all the one and the same run by an oligarchy. There are no food or drug or oil or banking or any other type of business. It is all the same run by the same people. If you go high enough on the ladder, you can see this. Average individual look around the supermarket and sees all kinds of different brands and thinks that there is a free market and competition between different companies. In reality, it is the scam designed to fool you so that you will think that. In reality, one food company can have 100 different brands. And different food companies can be owned by the same people that also own some other companies. These people can also be just partners to other people or just agents to their interest. Even if the same individuals or families do not own the different companies, these people work together. They even historically merry each other. Marriage is just another business arrangement for them. I will digress from food trade and look into one historical example that will show true aspect of Roman Empire economic and political system based on military, slavery, excess in food production, trade, and exploitation controlled by the elite that has been enforced on a global scale now.

During 17 and 18-century merchant families of Europe had made a fortune in far east trade. India had been conquered and colonized quite quickly, but China was a different story. Chinese people and state had been for a long time antagonistic to Europe and the west believing that all of the world evils have come from Europe. They had stuck to their own traditions and had closed country that did not enter into relations and trade with the west on the relevant scale. The big problem for the City of London merchants was how to pay for all of the goods that were coming from China. Chinese people and elite were not interested in any goods coming from Europe. They did not want to buy anything. At that time China was ruled by The Qing dynasty, and they had implemented extremely high taxes on European goods that had any form of acceptance in China. In the time that created a significant deficit in the City of London trade with China. Only one thing that was acceptable for trade and import to China was silver. The only thing that rulers of the Qing dynasty wanted to buy was silver and not all silver just one that is melted into bars. They did not want

European silver coins either. Great Britain did not have enough silver to pay for all of the tea, silk, and porcelain for which it had an enormous market in Europe, so they had to buy it with gold and gold-backed currencies. Price of silver went up, and so all of the prices of goods coming from China went up to. It created an inflationary spiral that slowly put Great Britain with all of its wars and expensive military into bid budget deficit. Rulers needed to find a solution to this problem. They needed to find something that they can trade for all of the goods coming from China. And eventually, they did. They find out one excellent agricultural product that they can sell. The product obtained from a poppy plant used in medicine from ancient times called opium. The Mediterranean region has the earliest archeological evidence of human use with the oldest known seeds that date back to more than 5000 BC in the Neolithic Age and had been used as food and as an anesthetic. In China, recreational use started in the 15th century but was restricted by its scarcity and price. Full blown opium ban in China began in 1729, yet was accompanied by nearly two centuries of ever-increasing opium use. The people had a hard life with extreme poverty, and one thing they liked that allowed them to escape from harsh reality was opium. Because opium was a hard addictive drug and once on it you became depended on constant use in a situation where you cannot afford it in extreme poverty your morals go away. Opium use usually comes with criminal behavior and hard structural Chinese society could not afford it. So it was banned.

British East India Company after a couple of wars gained the power to rule in India and to exercise a monopoly over opium production. To encourage slaves to cultivate the cash crops of indigo and opium with cash advances, and to prohibit the "hoarding" of rice they increase of the land tax to 50 percent of the value of crops doubling East India Company profits by 1777. That also created the Bengal famine of 1770. A genocide by starvation of 10 million people. Bengal opium was highly prized, and the illegal drug trade exploded. A number of addicts in China exploded, and trade deficit disappeared. Opium trade provided 15 to 20 percent of the entire British Empire's revenue and simultaneously caused scarcity of silver in China. The merchant families of Europe did a good business. The ship sailed full with British merchandise to India. Then they unloaded that and loaded opium for British-Chinese mafia network. In response, the Chinese Emperor took strong action to halt the import, including the seizure of cargo. Then the British navy came into the scene. British winning Hong Kong and trade concessions was a result. British ships sailed up through the Yangtze River and sank all of the smaller vessels that Chinese Emperor used for collecting tax, forcing the entire Chinese economy to collapse. Then France and USA forced China to give the same concessions to them also. China was later also forced by war to legalize opium and began massive domestic production. By 1906, the country was producing 85 percent of the world's opium, and the chunk of that was then exported to Indochina and other places. Most of us know this. We learn it in school. But what we did not learn in school was exactly what the school system does not want to teach you.

What were the names of people that owned East India Company? Who were the drug lords, and trade lords, and warlords and so on? What happened to their family fortune? It they controlled agriculture and world trade just 100 years ago, who inherit it and who controls it now? You see there is no trade. There is no food industry, or the drug industry or any other industry. It is trade, slavery, exploitation, war, hunger, genocide, politics, economy all in one and all the same. Power and control. Back in a day, the House of Sassoon handled the trading in opium and other goods in India. House of Jardine and Matheson handled distribution in China, and the House of Inchapes handled the shipping of these goods. House of Oppenheimer/Rhodes handled the gold and diamond mining business. The American operations were handled by the Sassoon, Jardine, Japhet and the House of Rockefeller. The House of Rothschild with Warburg as their agents coordinated the banking aspect of this trade. The House of Rothschild had the controlling share in the East Indian company too. Following Napoleon's defeat, they had acquired complete control over the entire British economy and presumably East India Company too. Nathan Mayer Rothschild was aware of the outcome of the Battle of Waterloo a full day before Wellington himself thanks to cartel intelligence network. Nathan controlling England funded Wellington's army, whereas James (Jacob), his own brother, operated out of France, funded Napoleon's army. It was war orchestrated by the same coffer and of course, being the first one informed of the result of the war Nathan began selling the consuls. It was designed in such a way that the selling on the market looked like as a sign of the British losing the battle, resulting in widespread panic in the markets and a vast panic sell-off was initiated. Nathan after initiating the selloff began secretly to acquire the consuls.

By the time word of the real situation of British victory came, the market rose up even higher than its previous levels, only this time most of it was already in Nathan hands with a return of approximately 20:1 on his investment making him the owner of almost entire British economy including East India Company. In 1815, Nathan Mayer made the following statement: "I care not what puppet is placed upon the throne of England to rule the Empire on which the sun never sets. The man who controls Britain's money supply controls the British Empire, and I control the British money supply." The business partnership of trading opium with China was also offered to the families that were the center of the new rising American oligarchy. That is how for example John Jacob Astor, got his opium trade business. His American Fur Company purchased ten tons of Turkish opium, then shipped the contraband item to Canton. All American families that were part of the opium trade had become an integral part of new American aristocracy with their leading partner in Europe. The Rothschild family and the City of London. In the US this trading cartel has even founded their own secret society at the Yale University. Internal circle of interest of this brotherhood was defended by a cartel of trading families like Taft, Russell, Bush, Rockefeller, Vanderbilt. Yale College itself was founded by Elihu Yale opium trader, slave trader and President of the East India Company settlement in Fort St. George, at Madras. Skull and Bones secret society was founded in 1832 by William Huntington Russell (cousin of Samuel Russell) and Alphonso Taft. The secret society's alumni organization, the Russell Trust Association, owns the society's real estate and oversees the organization. In 1823, Samuel Russell established Russell and Company for the purpose of acquiring opium in Turkey and smuggling it to China. Russell and Company bought out the Perkins(Boston) syndicate in 1830 and moved the primary center of American opium smuggling to Connecticut. Many of the European and American fortunes were made on the China (opium) trade. One of Russell and Company Chief of Operations, in Canton was Warren Delano Jr., grandfather of Franklin Roosevelt. Other Russell partners included Perkins, Sturgis, and Forbes, families. And they all did that with a permit of East India Company as a partner in trade. As a result of this Chinese society suffered total degradation. In 1906, 90 percent of people in Shanghai was addicted to heroin. Drugged from opium masses of people spent their days in opium dens in stupor incapable of any work.

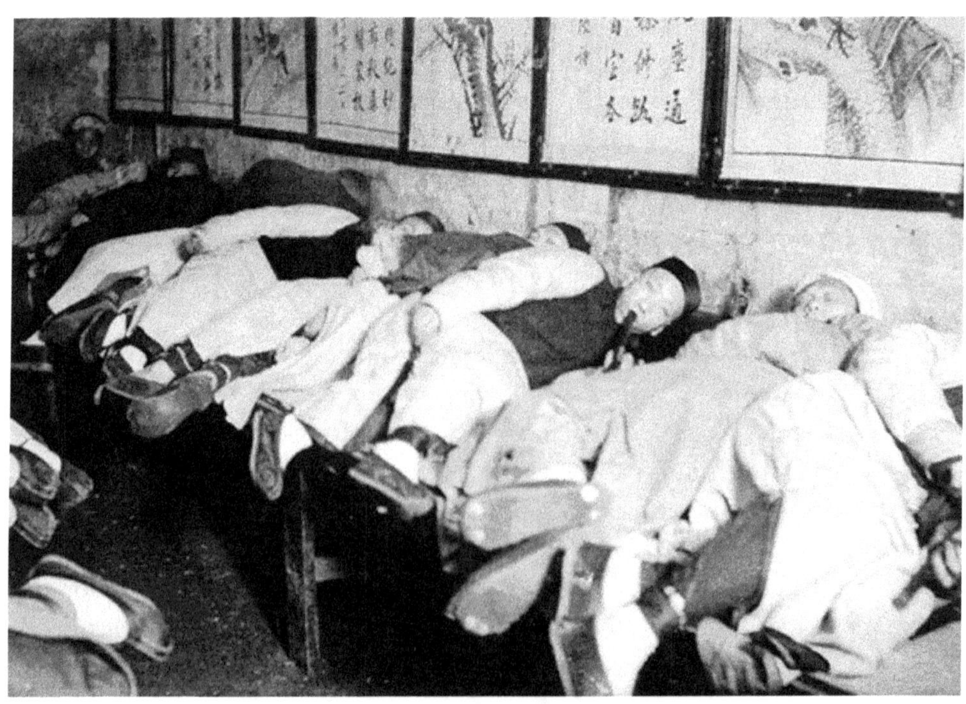

Trading in opium is technically drug trade like any other Big Pharma drug trade. The same people who made fortunes on drugs are the same people who make fortunes on cancer treatment drugs. The difference today is that we have synthetic heroin and your doctor prescribes it for cancer pains, and if you want to get something outside of "legal" business you will get jail sentence by the same people who made family fortunes on the opium trade back in the day. Under the Rockefeller drug laws, for example, the penalty for selling two ounces (57 g) of heroin, cocaine, or cannabis or possessing four ounces (113 g) or more of the same substances, was a minimum of 15 years to life in prison, and a maximum of 25 years to life in prison. The Rockefeller program drew intense opposition from civil rights advocates, who claimed that they were racist, as they were applied inordinately to African-Americans and, to a lesser extent, Latinos. One main criticism of these drug laws was that they put young minority males and females behind bars for carrying small amounts of drugs on them. In 2002, at age 46, Meile Rockefeller was arrested for protesting the Rockefeller drug laws. She was escorted by her brother, Stuart Rockefeller, and was backed by other members of the family including her grandfather's brother, Laurance Rockefeller. I can guess that some of the John spoiled brats did not learn the full extent of the Social Darwinism, but I am more inclined to think it is just "washing of the hands," we are not racist propaganda.

Today the six privately held grain companies were carved out from the centuries-old Mesopotamian-Roman-Venetian-Burgundian-Swiss-Amsterdam grain trade route, which today extends around the world. The "Big Six" grain cartel companies are New York-based Continental, Minneapolis-and Geneva-based Cargill; Paris-based Louis Dreyfus; São Paulo, Brazil- and the Netherlands, Antilles-based Bunge and Born; Lausanne, Switzerland-based André; and Illinois-and Hamburg, Germany-based Archer Daniels Midland/Töpfer. They issue no public stocks. They don't have an annual report. They are secretive as any bank, or government intelligence service. Two of these companies, Continental and Cargill, control 45-50% of the entire world's grain trade. Besides the grain ten to twelve pivotal companies, assisted by another three dozen, run the entire world's food supply. They are vital components of the Anglo-Dutch-Swiss food cartel, which is grouped around Britain's City of London. Cartel have complete control over entire world grains trade, the food and raw materials. But it also controls dairy, oil and fats, meat, fruits and vegetables, sugar, all forms of spices and so on. The entire world food trade and food production, and the processing and distribution, every aspect of it is controlled. These companies act even today as a food cartel. The oligarchy has developed four regions to be the principal world exporters of almost every type of food. These four regions are the European Union, especially Germany and France; the British Commonwealth nations of Canada, Australia, New Zealand, the Republic of South Africa; Argentina and Brazil in Ibero-America and the U.S. These four areas have a population of, at most 12% of the world's population. The rest of the world, with 88% of the population is dependent on the food exports from those regions. Every small country that has grain, dairy or other surpluses and wants to export them will encounter the problem. The cartel's four exporting regions were given monopoly in a brutal manner, with different regulations by the UN so that much of the rest of the world was thrust into enforced starvation.

If some of the other nations want to develop the oligarchy will not sell them seed for example, or fertilizer or any help in water management or any form of foreign investment would not be implemented. So when Chinese companies start to invest in this areas in Africa, for example, it turns into World War 3 because the oligarchy wants those regions under population control and any other form of control. They don't want for those regions to become self-sufficient so that they will depend on foreign aid and remain in the status of vassals states. Do as told and import or starve to death. At the same time Anglo-Dutch-Swiss food cartel is reducing the export regions self-sufficiency reducing the exporting countries like the US to a state of servitude as well. During the last couple of decades, millions of farmers in Argentina, Europe, Canada, US, Australia have also been destroyed by the same companies. For instance, in 1982, the US had 600,000 independent hog farmers. Today, that number is less than 150,000.

To average person five or six company to control entire world grain trade is hard to believe. But the real truth is that all of this companies work together. They are just one big cartel. They are not in competition. Every one of them has its part of the globe to control, and they coordinate their affairs with other ones and political-banking oligarchy. I will not analyze all of them but let us just look into biggest one so that we could have some idea how these things work. The biggest one is Cargill. It is founded shortly after the American Civil War by William Cargill, a Scottish immigrant and sea merchant. He bought his first grain elevator in Conover, Iowa. After that William Cargill expanded and bought grain elevators all along the Southern Minnesota Railroad, at a time when Minnesota was becoming an important shipping route. However, Cargill's largest break into the market was created when William purchased elevators along the line of James J. Hill's Great Northern railroad line. The line went west of Minneapolis, as far as North and South Dakota. Hill managed to do this because he was the business partner of Ned Harriman (father of Averell Harriman), who was the economic and business agent for Prince Edward, later King Edward VII. With a special rebate system and other arrangements, Hill's rail line helped build the Cargill operation. At that time Cargill was big but not part of the big oligarchy. It was just another bigger company like many others. Firm nearly went under twice. William Cargill, Jr., the son of company founder Will Cargill, made bad investments in Montana, and between 1909 and 1917, Cargill hovered on the brink of bankruptcy. What happened was that British capital came in to rescue the company. William Cargill had a daughter, Edna, who married John MacMillan. MacMillan family reorganize, pumped in the money and start to run the entire Cargill. John Hugh MacMillan II (1895-1960) was the director of Cargill from 1936 until 1957. He was also Knight Commander of Justice of the Sovereign Order of St. John. Secret society order controlled by the global aristocracy assorted around the Anglo-Dutch monarchy. Whitney MacMillan, chairman of Cargill from 1976 until 1994, was educated at the exclusive British-modeled Blake School (where the chairman of General Mills was also educated), and then Yale University. In another words, they were loyal to the oligarchy. Cargill also almost went under during the 1929 U.S. stock market crash, and the ensuing Great Depression. Only after that, the thing started to change. When you become part of the ruling system, you do not go bankrupt. You are too big to fail. It was still not big enough and what happened next is what defined Cargill as a "chosen one" to rule the food trade in America. There is nothing in history books of what was going on to Cargill Co. during the depression, 1865-1945. It is secret, but I managed to find out and we now know what happened. It was chosen to be saved by the oligarchy and used as a mechanism for control of the grain trade in one of the four regions.

One force came to the rescue: John D. Rockefeller's Chase National Bank, which sent its officer John Peterson to help run Cargill. Peterson became Cargill's top officer. Now if you are bankrupt and the big bank came with finances and rescue you and send people to run your company, then who really owns the company? You or the people that give you money from the bank? Then the way of conducting business of Cargill changed. It was not just one more regular let's make the business company. During the mid-1930s, Cargill started to use cut-throat tactics. In 1937, corn was a limited commodity. During 1936 crop had been a failure. Cargill purchased every possible corn future, to the tune of several millions of dollars, and organized a squeeze on the market. The Chicago Board of Trade directed Cargill to auction some of its futures to relieve the squeeze. Cargill refused and was expelled from the Board of Trade. The U.S. Secretary of Agriculture accused Cargill of trying to destroy the American corn market. And that is exactly what they wanted to do so that they can later buy it all with the help of the bank and create a control of the entire corn market. With the help of the Chase National Bank from the time of bankruptcy in the great depression, they started to expand globally in very short time. In 1953, Cargill set Tradax

International company in Panama to run its global grain trade. In 1956, it set up Tradax Genève, Switzerland. Thirty percent of Tradax is owned by old-line Venetian-Burgundian-Lombard banking families, particularly the Swiss-based Lombard, Odier, and Pictet banks. The investor for Tradax is the Geneva-based Crédit Suisse, which has been involved frequently in drug-money laundering. In 1985, the U.S. government accused Crédit Suisse and other large banks of laundering $1.2 billion in illegal drug money to the First National Bank of Boston. In 1977, Cargill's engagement in a "black peseta" laundering operation at Cargill's offices in Spain was also revealed. Cargill has been regularly cited for "blending" that is, adding foreign matter to its grain too. But it was chosen to be the controlling company of one part of the world food market by the ruling elite, and that is it. Today Cargill has expanded into every major crop and livestock on the face of the earth, in over 60 countries. It has also expanded into coal, steel, waste disposal, and metals and runs one of the 20 largest commodity brokerage firms in the United States, which is larger than most of the Wall Street brokerage houses.

When people talk about the food industry, they think Coca-Cola and Nestle. Coca-Cola and Nestle are not food industry. Far from it. Nestle is the biggest one on paper because oligarchy does not want regular people to know what is the real way of conducting business. That is the reason why, by design these companies like Cargill and others issue no public stock or annual report. It is only truthful to say that we do not know which one is the biggest, and it is not Nestle for sure. Again as I written before these companies are more secretive than any oil company, bank, or government intelligence service. However, even stupid Coca-Cola have the same pattern of behavior.

If you want to know what is the secret ingredient to Cola syrup, I will tell you. It is Nazi Germany. The story of Coca-Cola begun with an alcoholic beverage called Pemberton's French Wine Cola created by druggist John Stith Pemberton who was also morphine addict too.

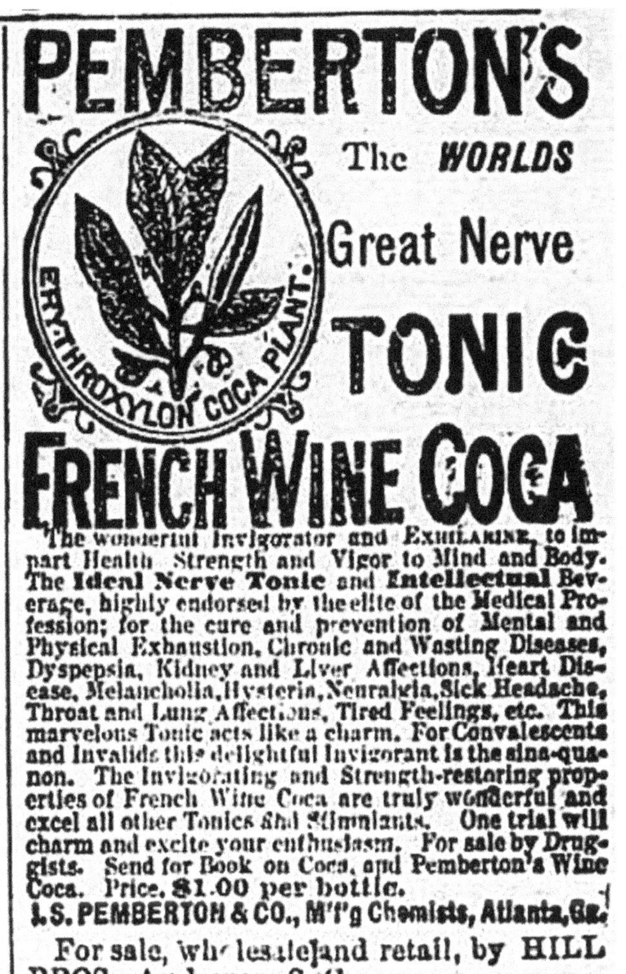

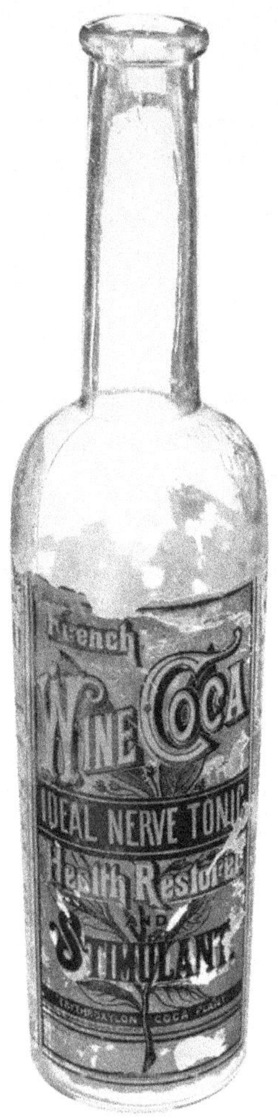

Among its ingredients was a euphoria-inducing mixture of alcohol and cocaine called cocaethylene. The drink marketed as a sexual stimulant and "a most wonderful invigorator of sexual organs" was outlawed following new temperance laws in 1885. Pemberton replaced wine with sugar syrup and debuted new product in 1886. It was marketed as "ideal brain tonic." Coca-Cola remained cocaine infused until 1903 when the company bowed to white fears of exploding cocaine use among African Americans. As a story goes African Americans have taken to "sniffing" since deprived of Whisky by prohibition as a "new southern menace." Because of the Coca-Cola, African Americans had been gained access to the cocaine in increasing numbers because beverage became cheap and was sold for a nickel each with the introduction of bottles in

1899. However, it took some more time and Coca-Cola everywhere became completely cocaine-free by 1929 but was still infused and it is infused to this day by coca leaf extract for taste purposes.

Coca-Cola is the only company in the world, well actually Stepan Company the different one, but for the interest of making Coca-Cola is the only company allowed by the government to import and process coca leaves. Stepan Company import leaves mostly from South America from countries like Peru and Columbia. And it is all legal. If Coke can work partnerships to bring coca leaves into the United States, why can't the rest of us? Are there different laws for different people? If I were to travel to Peru and try to go to the US with a small batch of coca leaves (perhaps to brew tea), I would be detained by border officials. Coke has no doubt liked it this way because competition for coca leaves would drive up prices, which is never good for business. If you really want to know why is cocaine the most expensive drug on the black market it is because of Coca-Cola which needs hundreds of tons of leaves annually. A syrup is only made in the US and then shipped worldwide because it is "secret ingredient." How is it possible that generic 7-up or grape soda, for example, can fool our taste buds, yet finding a generic cola capable of mimicking the awesomeness that is Coke remains all but impossible? That is Cola secret ingredient. The crazy reason why no company can truly emulate the taste of Coke. Because coca leaf extract as an ingredient no other company in the world can bye. And doing business with Guatemalan death squads to kill union leaders in late 70s and pioneering the supersizing of America is just added bonus.

In 2001, a lawsuit was filed on behalf of the Colombian labor union Sinaltrainal (National Union of Food Workers) in the Florida Third District Court of Appeal, demanding a monetary compensation for $500 million for the deaths of nine workers, members of the National Union for Food Industry Workers who worked in the Coca-Cola Bebidas y Alimentos plant in Carepa in northern Colombia. Like Guatemalan "incident" was not enough. They accused Coca-Cola and its Colombian bottling partners of using paramilitary death squads to murder, torture and kidnap labor union leaders. The suit alleged that company hired militants of the United Self Defense Forces of Columbia (AUC) to murder nine union members including Isidro Segundo Gil who was shot dead inside Coca-Cola plant. The physical access the paramilitaries have had to bottle plants is impossible without company knowledge because all of the Coca-Cola plants have cameras and private security. Federal Judge Jose E. Martinez progressed the case forward against two Coca-Cola bottlers: Bebidas y Alimentos and Pan-American Beverages, but not against Coke itself. Judge Martinez later dismissed the remaining claims against the two bottlers partly because the Colombian bottling plants were not owned by Coca-Cola company.

PR folks that are in charge do not want their brand name tarnished, so they like to confuse the topic in any way. Coca-Cola says that assassinations of the Colombian union members are not its responsibility because they are not employed by Coca-Cola directly. The reason why Coca-Cola have other companies bottling the product around different countries around the world is exactly this. They are giving up some small cut from the profits in exchange for plausible deniability. Well-designed strategy. They do not want to be dragged in courts if something happens, and it is not really question about money for them. It is about brand image and marketing. They are selling the dream. Even the red Santa Claus is their invention. Some research and brain scans have found that for example when Americans travel, and they do not feel safe in some third world country. When they see Coca-Cola sign, it has a soothing effect on them. It is because from an early age they had been a condition to associate good feelings with the symbol of Coke. Coca-Cola itself was found to have done extensive research into something called neuromarketing. Marketing people like to call it "buy button." Subconsciously condition behavior through association. It has never been the case that you were just drinking sugary fuzzy fluid named Coke. The flavor and the perception of it is a composite perception that your brain builds out of a lot of pieces of things including the emotions that are associated subconsciously with the brand message and other things that brand message has been associated with. Brands actually have a taste.

In reality violence, abuse and exploitation leveled against Coke workers and communities have been uncovered in many other countries as well, notably China, El Salvador, Guatemala, India, Mexico, and Turkey. In extension to the exploitation of workers, Coke has been implicated in the exploitation of children by profiting from hazardous child labor in sugar cane fields in El Salvador and sucking all the underground waters in India creating a catastrophe for local villagers. It takes two liters of water to create one liter of Coca-Cola. In 2004 Human Rights Watch said that if Coca-Cola wanted to avoid complicity in child labor, it should recognize its responsibility to respect human rights. Above all Coca-Cola is about image and it is going to spend more than two billion dollars on marketing to convince you "life tastes good." Thanks in part to Coca-Cola marketing campaigns the supersizing of the American obesity problem and its bottom line led to a situation where sugary nutrition devoid sodas are one of the main sources of calories in the American diet. In America, more than 80 percent of death-row inmates are requesting Coke for their last meal. Also when you market soft drinks that contain caffeine like Coca-Cola to young children you are getting them addicted to the stimulants early on. Caffeine (that is neurotoxin) can have a detrimental effect on childhood brain development. It is not just the question of obesity. Every 330 ml can of Coke has 34.5 mg of caffeine and diet Coca-Colas have even more. That is enough to stimulate dopamine release in the brain and create cravings and alter behavior in adults but give Cola to children they will become hyperactive and addicted. The brains of children have greater sensitivity to caffeine effects than the brains of adults. Caffeine can cause them to be hyperactive immediately after drinking it, which is obvious and there is too much of refined sugar in the coke as well giving them a burst of energy. However, it also can make them nervous, anxious, worsen stomach problems and create sleep problems in the long run. The evidence does not show that caffeine stunts growth, but it can make them addicted to it. What happens is the same thing that happens in adults. In cases of daily use of Coca-Cola infused with caffeine brain compensate in expectation of toxin and until child drinks it is having brain fog, low energy, attention problems and can be nervous. Same like any other drug addict addicted to amphetamines. If someone has a predisposition to anxiety, it can agitate the situation by creating neurotic type behavior and chronic stress. Children that have attention difficulties like ADD (Attention-Deficit Disorder) and attention deficit hyperactivity disorder (ADHD) should avoid any stimulants like caffeine. Combination of caffeine, sugar and excitotoxins like aspartame and monosodium glutamate (MSG) can exuberate symptoms in children that are already on the ADD side into full-blown illness. Then the child would be prescribed the real amphetamine-based drug called Ritalin. Children will suffer withdrawal effects just like adults if they do not have it, at the very least a headache. It is a serious public health issue.

To increase the problem of these caffeinated drinks is the fact that many of them are full with sugar. That is bad nutrition. If you have a child that is drinking more than one sugary drink per day, the child is a set-up for obesity. Because there is no fiber to slow down digestion blood sugar will spike rapidly, and then it will crash creating hypoglycemia. And the child will seek another Coke. The earlier your child's brain is addicted to stimulants like caffeine and refined sugar the earlier obesity will begin and the more likely it is to follow you into adulthood. And the industry loves it. Drinking sugary caffeinated drinks is habit-forming. It is very clever to put caffeine in a sugary drink and then market that drink to children.

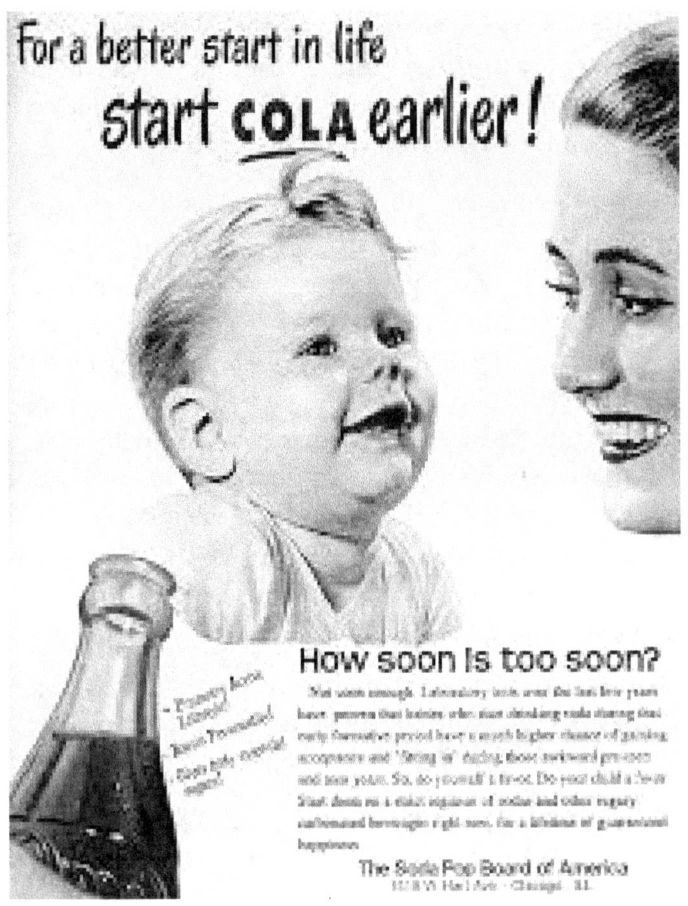

Also given the research that has been conducted in animal models (Horger et al., 1991; Schenk et al., 1994), it is possible that habitual caffeine use may lead to cross-sensitization of the neural reward substrate to illicit drugs which is a problem beyond obesity. If you give Coke to your children, then don't just believe me, do your own research and see what is truth. You can read this review if you want (Caffeine Use in Children: What we know, what we have left to learn, and why we should worry Neurosci Biobehav Rev. 2009 Jun; 33(6): 793–806. doi: 10.1016/j.neubiorev.2009.01.001). Do we think that Coca-Cola does not know this? Caffeine was always in the formula, not "just" cocaine. Two basic ingredients that are engraved in Coca-Cola name are Coca leaves and Cola nut. Cola nut contains caffeine. When they kick out cocaine, they kept in the formula the second best legal stimulant drug that they can use, caffeine. Coca-Cola claims that caffeine is an integral part of its complex flavor, but that is a lie. Caffeine does not have a taste. We cannot distinguish between caffeinated and noncaffeinated drinks. It is there for modification of consumer behavior. Coca-Cola once said that capturing a high school consumer meant keeping them for 50 to 60 years. Their real target that they want to "capture" is actually children. Coca-Cola wants to buy a world of Coke and why? Well, they say they want to spread the peace, love, and brotherhood to everyone.

However, they actually used World War 2 to establish dominance on a global market. After the attack on Perl Harbor at the US government's expanse, meaning taxpayer money, Coke employees were dressed up in army uniforms and given completely made up the name of "technical observers." Then they were sent around the world to establish 64 bottling plants behind the lines. This action plan positioned them to expand and take the entire markets and became monopolists in all war-devastated economies. With the help of the US military, they expanded to become the global leader in soft drink production soon after the WW2. Today you can be anywhere on the planet except for North Korea and Cuba and get a Coke just around the corner even in places where there is no clean drinking water or electricity. Coca-Cola also had no problem with Nazis. It was one of the three official beverage sponsors of the 1936 Summer Olympics in Berlin.

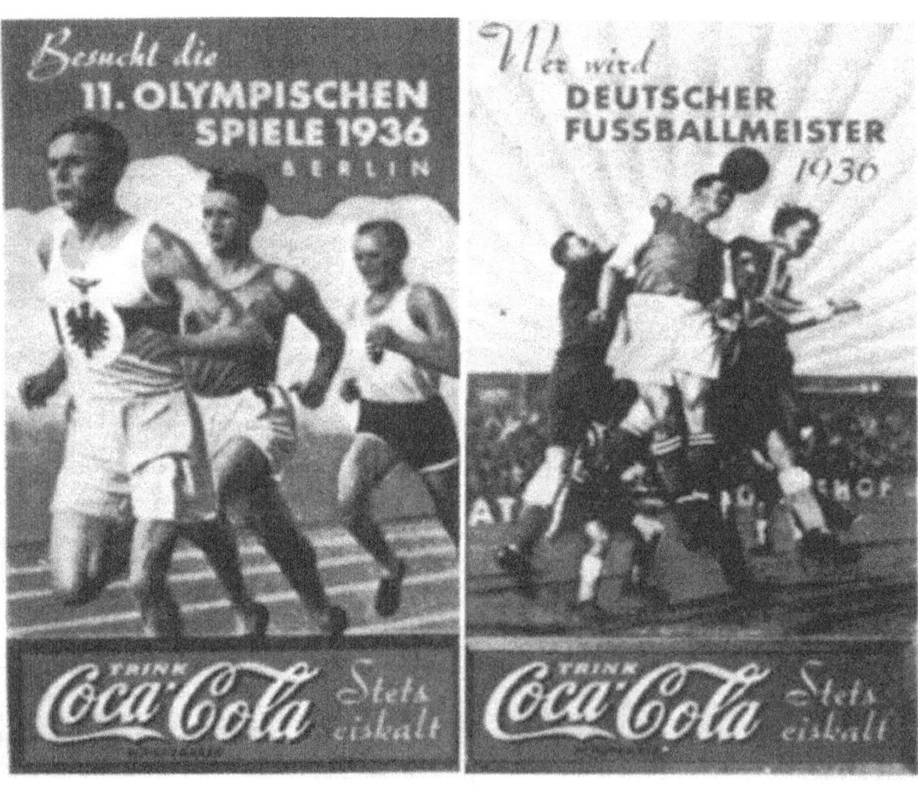

Advertising and bottling and expanding rapidly to cover the entire Germany market under Hitler. Corporations from America rebuild Germany after the WW2 and supported the early Nazi regime and then when the war broke out they figured out the way to keep their business going. General Motor was able to keep Opel (100 percent GM-owned subsidiary) and continue to make basically most of the Germany tanks that were used in war. It was American company actually that made all tanks and arm vehicles that Hitler solders drove. General Motors was notably more significant to the Nazi war machine than Switzerland. "Enemy" was driving trucks manufactured by Ford and Opel and flying Opel-built warplanes. Again Opel was 100 percent GM-owned subsidiary. Ford was able to keep its thing going. We already know about Standard Oil and IG Farben. They kept their thing going. IBM was able to keep its thing going and continue to produce computers for death camps. Nazis used them in Auschwitz and other places to track Jew inmates (Hollerith punch card machine look more like type machine then computer). By request from Nazis, IBM invented the national census. Thousands of people were hired by IBM, put into the giant warehouse. People went door to door, filled out census forms including religion and residence. All of this information was punched in to punch cards. All the banks also used IBM punch cards, so confiscation of the property and business was a piece of cake. Auschwitz tattoo is IBM number. IBM also developed a special program by request from the Nazi regime by which all of the skills were put into one set of cards so that they could cross-tabulate that against where slave labor is needed so that they can work prisoners to death before the gas chamber. However, what about companies like Coca-Cola. Because they needed their "secret ingredient" in the form of coca leaf extract, they could not keep their thing going. So what they did was they invented a new drink that they can produce with local ingredients made in Germany. That drink was Fanta Orange for the Germans. Named Fanta from the German word for fantastic. At the time when the Nazis came to power in 1933, Coca-Cola's business in Germany was already booming. The direction of a man named Max Keith has helped the company adapt and expend under the Nazi regime. He renewed the Coca-Cola brand in the country and boosted sales even before the Nazi regime. Cola was well known and accepted drink as much as it was in the US. By the time Adolf Hitler ascended to the proverbial throne in 1933 sales of Coca-Cola had risen from 6,000 cases a year to 100,000. When Nazis came to power, it was no problem for Cola to do business with them too. They have no problem with Nazi racist ideology what so ever as long as they can make a lot of sales. Through the 1936 Berlin Olympic games, for example, Keith secured that attendants had all the Coke they could want. However, the Coca-Cola Company's interests were hurt later that year when the Nazi regime began to seriously restrict imports from foreign nations to protect the German economy, and on the list was Coca-Cola syrup to as a non-German product.

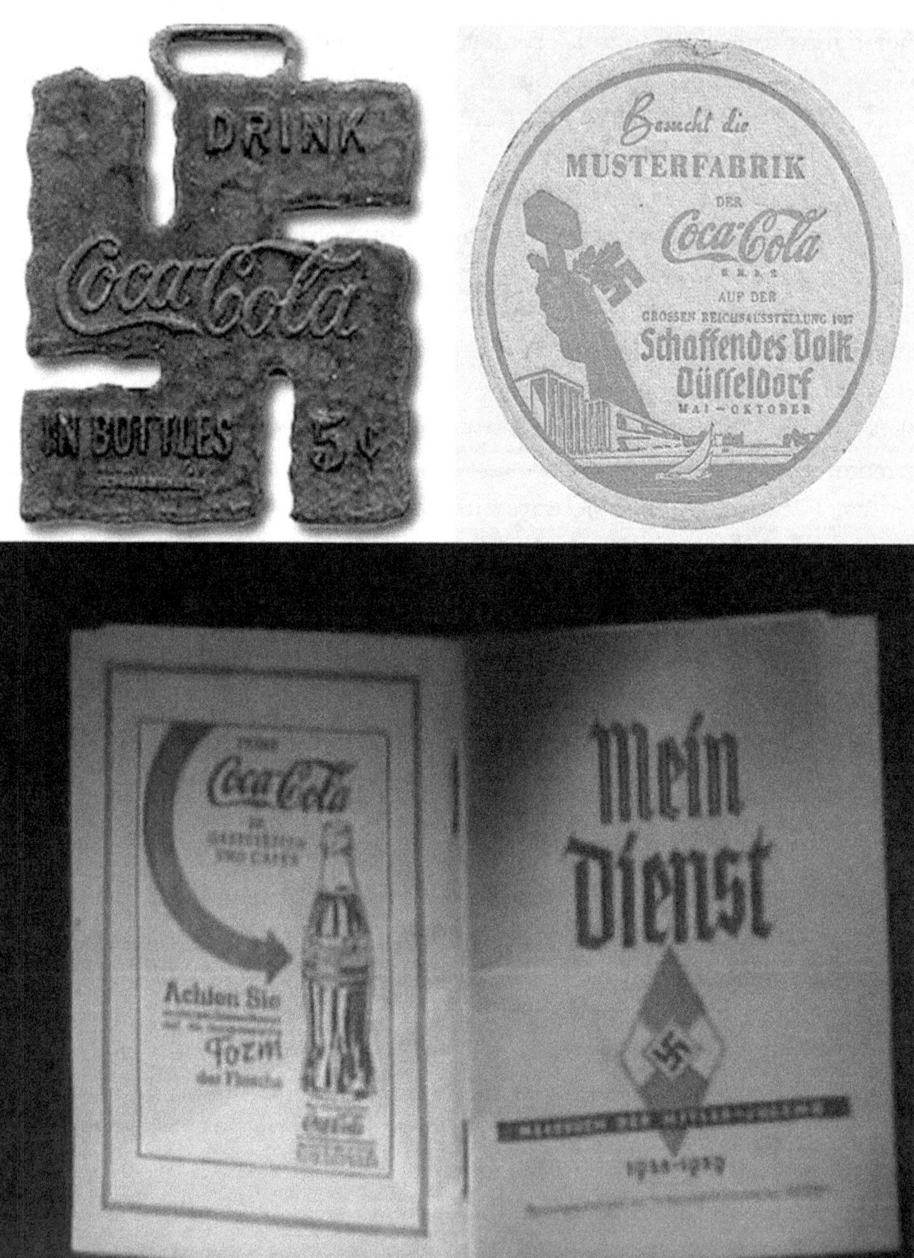

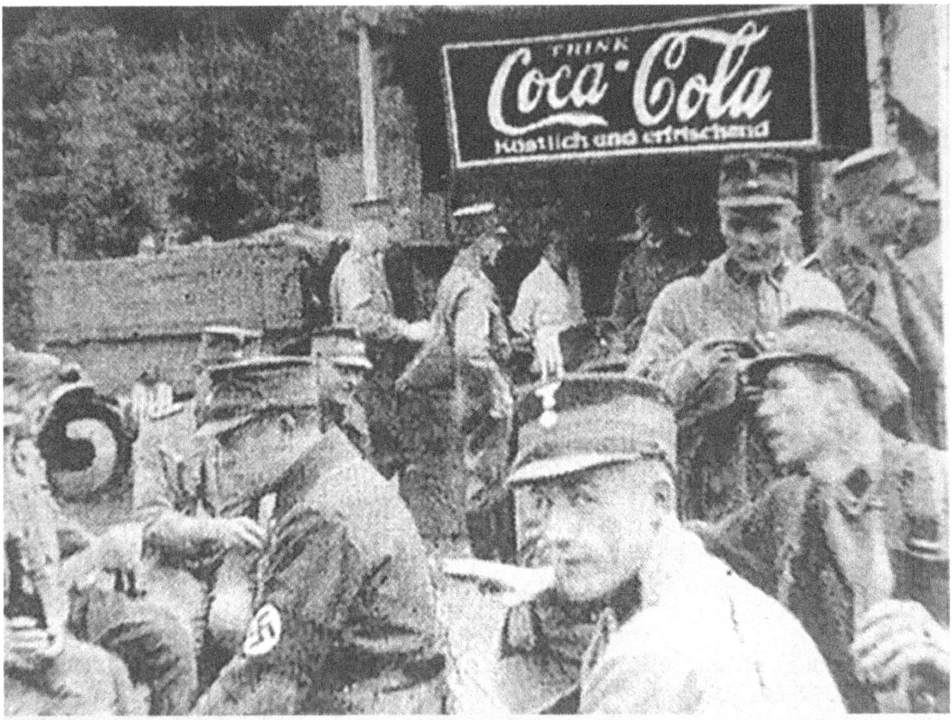

THINK
Coca-Cola
köstlich und erfrischend

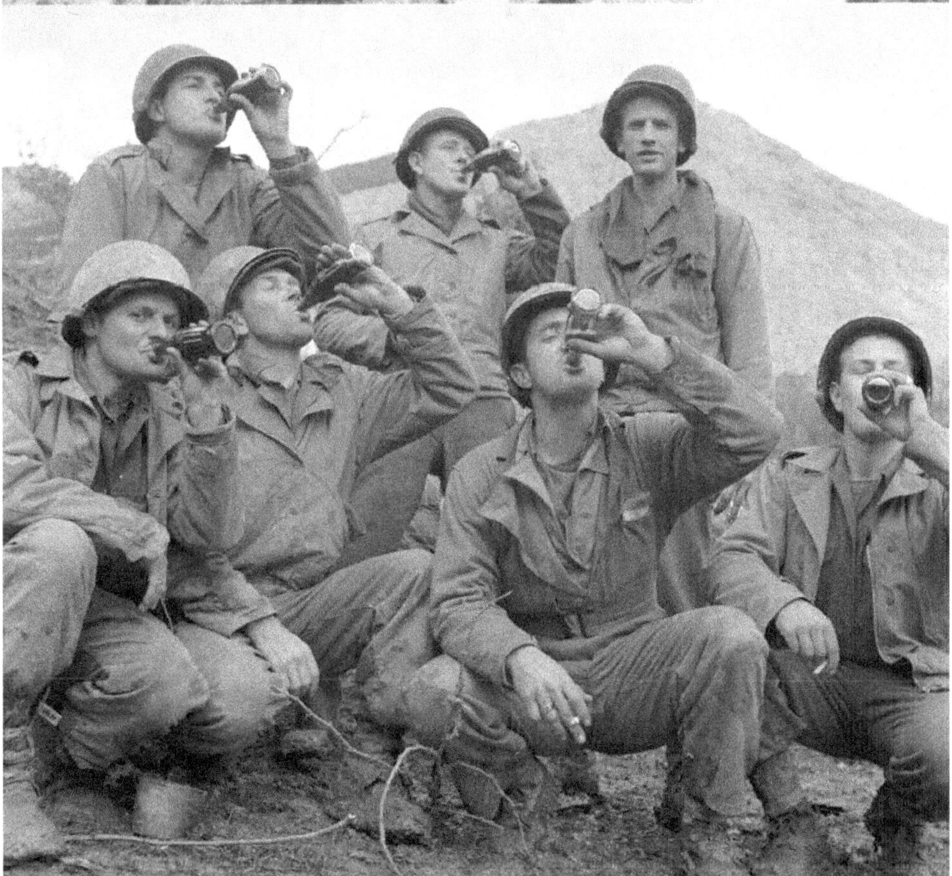

However, the director of the Coca-Cola Company communicated by a third party to convince Hermann Göring, Hitler's second in command, to allow the importation of this syrup. At this point, Cola was dealing directly with the Nazis politically. Advertising campaign worked to convince the beer drinking populace that fizzy drinks were good alternative for the workingman while on job and slogans urged the industrial labor force to down tools and drank a refreshing bottle of Coca-Cola.

When propaganda minister Joseph Goebbels booked out the Sportpalast for mass displays of rhetoric, Coca-Cola billboards appeared outside, right where the party faithful were queuing. Not long after, in 1937, Coca-Cola took an extra hit in their attempts to sell their products in Germany when a German official at a rival soda company, Afri-Cola, began distributing pictures of Coke bottle tops from the US that showed the Hebrew characters identifying it as Kosher. They used this as evidence to claim that a Jew secretly ran the Coca-Cola Company. A Bavarian spring-water bottler suffering from loss of profits got in on the act too, writing to the Food and Agriculture Ministry in Berlin to opine that: "It would be interesting to know whether Jewish capital is active in Coca-Cola GmbH." Sales tanked, and the Nazi HQ canceled their orders, forcing Keith to deny any Jewish connection in an advert placed in the Party's propaganda sheet, Der Stuermer. To counteract this notion further, and the ensuing loss of profits from German consumers, Keith began to brand the Coca-Cola Company in Germany as pro-Nazi aggressively. At one Nazi convention, at the celebration Keith ordered a mass "Sieg Heil" in honor of Hitler's 50th birthday, to commemorate: "Our deepest admiration and gratitude for our Führer who has led our nation into a brilliant higher sphere." He also reached out specifically to target the Hitler Youth, attempting to win over the younger generation of Nazis as a standard Coca-Cola policy of marketing to children in order to get them addicted in the young age. At one occasion in the Reichsausstellung Schaffendes Volk in Dusseldorf, an exhibition that celebrated the achievements of the German worker under the Nazi regime, Coca-Cola wormed its way into the floorplan of this propaganda-fest with a miniature train for the children, a model bottling plant that could wash, cap and fill 4,000 bottles an hour and a 16-metre (50-foot)-long service counter selling ice-cold Cokes to the stupefied punters. Amid the spectacle, Hermann Göring himself paused to enjoy a cool glass of the brown stuff, a moment captured by a company photographer. With war developed in Europe, Keith worried that his foreign-linked business could be nationalized and that he will be thrown in jail. With his connections in the Third Reich, he was appointed a supervisor of all soft-drink factories in Germany and all of its conquered territories. He soon managed the company in Italy, France, Holland, Luxembourg, Belgium, and Norway. At the time, Coke sold around 4.5 million cases annually in Nazi Germany. However, in 1940, as World War 2 advanced, Keith started to worry on import limitations. Out of concern, he produced a new syrup from local ingredients to be used if they could not get access to the official Coca-Cola syrup from America. To conjure up a new drink they used homegrown apple fibers left over from the cider-making process and whey. At first, with a dwindling supply of Coca-Cola, Keith worked to ensure that his sodas only went to hospitals to wounded soldiers who were particularly members of the Nazi Party. When they had completely run out of Coca-Cola, the company started selling Fanta, which was a smash hit among the German populace. In 1941, Keith used his political connections to get around the ban on sugar. Fanta tasted better than rival drinks and became very popular. Housewives even flavored soups and stews with it. It sold 3 million cases in 1943. When the war ended in 1945, "technical observers" took over the administration of German industry. Keith embraced the T.O.s, but they declined to employ him, with one calling him "a second Hitler." The Coca-Cola Company got back control of their German division and, despite being ousted by the occupying U.S. military as Nazi collaborators, Woodruff reinstated Keith. He was praised as a hero by the Americans back in Atlanta for keeping the company alive in Germany.

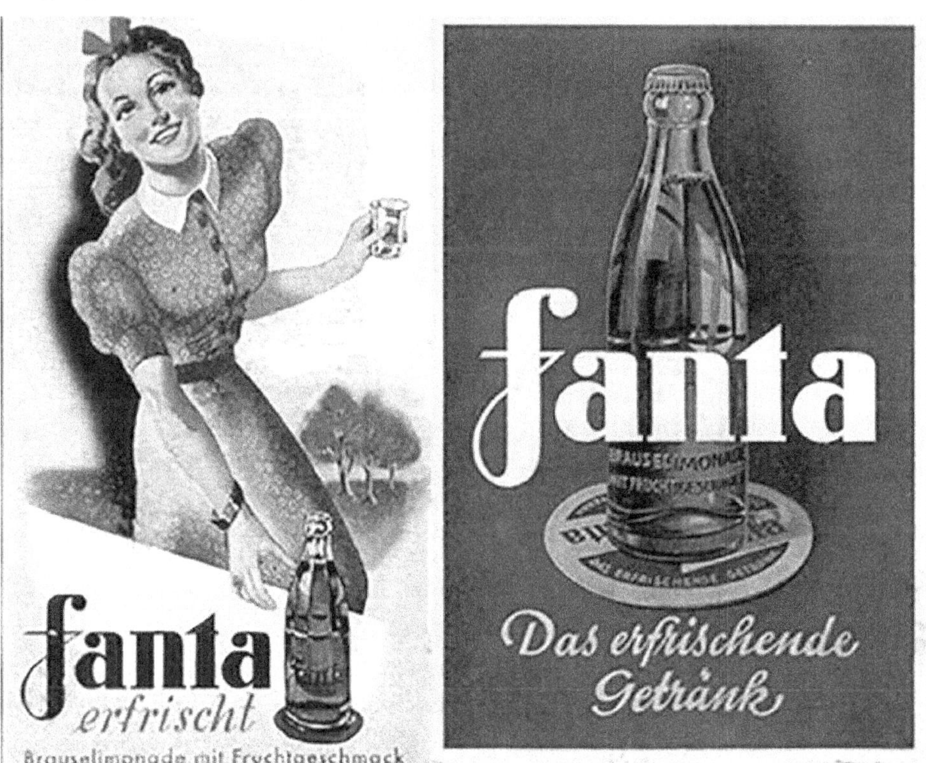

The company's VP of Sales, Harrison Jones, praised Keith by calling him a "great man" for operating in dire circumstances. He was actually rewarded for all of the good work for Coca-Cola, eventually naming him Coca-Cola's chief for all

Europe (Some rebellious bottlers referred to him as "Super-Führer"). The production of Coca-Cola was quickly reestablished, and Fanta was discontinued for the time being. In April 1955, Coca-Cola reintroduced Fanta with a new recipe, this time as an orange-flavored drink. They revived the name largely because it was convenient. Coca-Cola already had the copyright, and I think they thought no one would pay attention to history. They will not mention this, one word of this, in World of Coca-Cola museum. When you ask them, PR folks of Coca-Cola today and for example fake-truth facts-sites like Snopes will tell you that real fact-check truth is that: "Fanta was the creation of a German-born Coca-Cola man who was acting without direction from Atlanta." This is a quote from Snoopes.com that "has long been engaged in the battle against misinformation."

Now, do we think that the US Government did not know about all of this? Of course, they did. US Government is the largest consumer of IBM products for example. It is the same system. Democracy is a story for the public. Deep state and Federal Reserve (privately owned reserve) run things like economy and geopolitics. Sometimes US Government may even decide to run some experiments on American people without consent as they did in Tuskegee syphilis experiment for example. The secret experiment conducted by the U.S. Public Health Service. The purpose of this study was to observe the natural progression of untreated syphilis in rural African-American men in Alabama under the guise of receiving free health care from the United States government. They wanted to know how fast the diseases can spread in population for their military bioweapon programs and if there is a need for population reduction. It was not experiment about syphilis as many people believe. Hundreds of men, all black and poor signed up. Some of the men assumed they are being treated for rheumatism or bad stomachs. They were promised free physicals, free meals, and free burial insurance. The researchers never received knowledgeable permission from the men and never told the men with syphilis that they were not being treated but were simply being observed until they died and their bodies examined for ravages of the disease. US government kills. Sometimes they kill their own citizens with diseases. Well, they will deny this by saying that 431 men, all of them had previously contracted syphilis before the study began and that 169 that did not have it where chosen for the control group. The government will say that the men were given free medical care, meals, and free burial insurance for participating in the study. And all of this is just a lie. Firstly, the men were told that the study was only going to last six months, but it actually lasted 40 years. Initially, when the investigation began, treatment for syphilis was not effective, often dangerous and fatal. However, even after penicillin was discovered and used as a treatment for the disease, the men in the Tuskegee study were not offered the antibiotic. They were used in the same manner that prisoners of WW2 where used in death caps with one exception. These men did not know that they were used. We as the public will never have known about all of this.

In 1966, a public health service inspector had some issues about the study. Peter Buxtun wrote to the executive of the U.S. Division of Venereal Diseases about the ethics of the experiment. However, the agency ignored Buxtun's concerns. Buxtun eventually got angry and leaked a report about the study to an Associated Press journalist named Jean Heller, who years later termed it: "One of the grossest violations of human rights I can imagine." On July 26, 1972, Heller's story appeared on the front page of the New York Times, revealing that the men had deliberately been left untreated for 40 years. And one big question remains. How many of such experiments are still out there that nobody had leaked? Fort Detrick in it times employed some 300 scientists including 140 micro-biologists, 40 of whom had PhDs, 250 specialists from different disciplines and around 700 to 1000 supporting staff. It produced some 900,000 mice, 50,000 guinea pigs, 2,500 rabbits, and 4,000 monkeys annually. Publicly U.S. government acknowledge only weaponizing seven viruses. However, what some evidence shows there are actually hundreds of them if we count all of the weaponized cancer viruses, and other "not instantly lethal" ones. By the documents that are available the list of viruses experiment on contains cancer, leukemia, lymphoma, sarcoma, encephalitis, herpes, influenza, mononucleosis, as well as prions that cause mad cow disease and hundreds of others.

Now, why would someone want to weaponized sv40 cancer virus? It is not instantly lethal. It cannot affect any military conflict scenario. The only consequence of using weaponized cancer viruses will be a higher mortality rate of cancer in the prolonged time period leading to a higher overall mortality rate. The weaponized cancer viruses are hard to detect and only can be effective as some sort of population reduction mechanism. The year after Fort Detrick was publicly closed DoD's biological weapons budget actually rise from $21,9 to $23,2 million. They got even more money to research "defensive" instead "offensive" bioweapons. Even the stockpiled biological weapons that were pledged to be destroyed remained in tacked in Pine Bluff, Arkansas. The focus on weapons of mass destruction focused from the atomic bomb to a single mutated strain of engineered viruses and then after that to the realm of immunological attack. Using cancer viruses manufactured in labs featured a new field called retrovirology that also included the production of aids like the immunosuppressive type of new virus strains. Ebola-like immune system destroyers for both warfare and population control.

Fort Detrick had become a headquarters for the National Cancer Institute after the so-called ending of a biological weapons program. Company Lytton

Bionetics operated the entire administration of the National Cancer Institute programs at Fort Detrick at that time. This private company was a medical subsidiary of the mega military weapons contractor called Litten Industries. Litton president Roy Ashe was Nixon alternate for the National Security Adviser post he gave to Kissinger and went to join the White House staff. Kissinger immediately ordered the assessment of America biological weapons capability and agreed to pursue the less destructive option of Ebola-like viruses, and the contract went to his White House company friends Litton Bionetics. So the private companies in collusion with the government had continued the bioweapons program. This group of people at Bionetics combined leukemia, lymphoma and sarcoma viruses to create new type ones that human biology does not have the immune system defense. The researchers had fined for example document named National cancer institute number 71-2025 titled "Investigations of viral carcinogenesis in primates" in which there where commutation of numerous type of viruses. Experimenting with sv40 cancer viruses is big taboo to this day. Nobody ever wants to touch the subject. They always conveniently talk about anthrax or some deadly germ when someone mentions biological weapons and agents. There was even one incident with vaccines. Initial hepatitis b vaccines were manufactured in contaminated chimpanzees supplied by Merc the US military leading biological weapons contractor. New York city gay men injected with them between 1972 and 1974 developed AIDS. Litton Bionetics that supplied Merc company African green monkeys that were discovered to be a source of the pandemic of AIDS virus from Africa. They did not know or didn't want to test for AIDS at that time. Lytton Bionetics supplied Merc drug company with contaminated chimpanzees from which the first hepatitis b vaccines were prepared for trials in New Your city on gay men. Additional test subjects for this mission included Willowbrook state school developmentally disabled children on Staten Island and sex workers and health professionals in Central Africa and Haiti. Outside US the Soviet Union did extensive research into germ warfare too. What is conclusion from all of this. Experimenting with sv40 cancer viruses and other non-instantly lethal microorganisms by U.S. government is big taboo to this day. Weaponizing cancer viruses was continued by the private companies after Fort Detrick was closed as bioweapon programs that are part of Pig Pharma and paid by taxpayers money. The same Big Pharma that supposedly are also researching the cure for cancer. By now you should understand what this means and what is the philosophy of eugenics.

One more interesting topic is why U.S. government is poisoning water deliberately by adding fluoride. We all know it is a toxin, and other less toxic chemicals can do the same thing, but the fluoride is the chemical of choice. Why? It affects the human brain, but that is not the main reason. Siberian gulags and

Nazi death camps did use it for this effect on human mental state. It is hazardous waste from phosphate fertilizer industry which cannot be dumped into the sea by international law and cannot be used locally because it is too concentrated. So government to save money for the industry just dumps it to the drinking water. Effect on the human mental state is just added bonus. Today most countries do not fluoridate. According to the WHO data tooth decay in 12-year-olds is coming down as fast in both fluoridated and non-fluoridated countries. It is not about tooth decay. Never were. It is just the scam for justification. A way for industry and government to fool you. By 1930 aluminum industry among others was the biggest pollutant of fluoride. In that time both deaths of people and animals from fluoride toxic fumes and pollution was common. The only one company in America doing aluminum business was Alcoa (from Aluminum Company of America). At that time U.S. public health service was under direct jurisdiction of U.S. Secretary of the Treasury Andrew William Mellon. The son of banker Thomas Mellon, owner of the family banking business, T. Mellon & Sons, also branched out into other businesses. Mellon helped finance the establishment of Alcoa and was a major stockholder. By the 1920s, he was one of the richest people in the country, paying more in income taxes than all but two other American industrialists. He was also the founder of Mellon Institute of Industrial Research. Founded in 1913 and merged lather with the Carnegie Institute of Technology in 1967 to form Carnegie Mellon University in Pittsburgh, Pennsylvania, United States.

This institute was notorious for founding research that gives industry the scientific backing for defending itself and pushing their goals. Mellon Institute was the one that published some of the key studies that provided evidence that fluoride is good at fighting teeth decay. What was the most probable scenario was that they did wide range of studies from many different fields until they discovered one possible application of what was known until that time just as heavy nerve toxin and rat poison. It was doctor Dr. Gerald Cox who was hired and was working for the Mellon Institute that made the first proposal to fluoridate public water supplies artificially. Not much longer after that official human experiment began in January of 1945 just after WW2. Another part of the story is that, during the Second World War, industrial fluoride pollution increased because of the production and extensive use of Alcoa aluminum in aircraft construction. It was after the World War 2 that several governments began to put fluoride in water supplies to protect people against cavities because there where large quantities of the toxic waste that cannot be put in rivers or anywhere else. Disposal of such large scale would cost billions and will mean environmental disaster. People at that time unlike now know very well what rat poison actually is. Early "conspiracy theorists" declared that it was all just a communist scheme to undermine American public health.

A common argument from a moral and ethical view was that the public has not chosen to be consuming it and so it is against individual will. There are other ways to fight tooth decay. One will be just to don't eat sugar. Who brush the teeth of monkeys? Did they or other animals in the wild have such high-level dental plan as we do? There are even other chemicals that also fight bacteria without being on the same level of toxicity. Chlorine is put into the public pools to fight infections and in water supply in Europe not to fight tooth decay but to disinfect water. Chlorine itself is highly toxic. In the U.S. there must be an organization that has invested interest in using fluoride otherwise it would not be going into the water the way that it is. Fluoride is not just a key ingredient for making aluminum. It is used for making steel. It is used for producing high-octane gasoline. The Manhattan Project needed fluoride to enrich uranium. The biggest industrial building in the world, for a time, was the fluoride gaseous diffusion plant in Tennessee in the Manhattan Project. If workers realized that the fluoride they were breathing is causing injury to them, the Manhattan Project would be jeopardized because there were be a lot of lawsuits from workers. And even more from farmers living around these industrial plants. Sodium fluoride from the aluminum industry was the most common pollutant in the early stages, but today the industry had shifted, and there is another type of fluoride that is the most common.

Today it is the fluoride acid (hydrofluorosilicic acid), that comes from phosphate fertilizer industry. It is a byproduct, a toxic waste. The fluoride bound to silica (sand) is one of the most corrosive acids out there. It can eat through concrete, stainless steel, glass, fiberglass, plastic, you name it, and it would eat it. Today even in China the fluoridation of the water is forbidden by law. No baby fluoridated water in China. They sell to the U.S. most of their stockpiles of this toxic fluoride waste. When you dig up rocks that are used in the phosphate fertilizer industry, they are no good in that state. You have to mix them with sulphuric acid, and this reaction produces soluble phosphate and hydrofluorosilicic acid. So you see. It is a good strategy. These people are smart. Today they are making billions of dollars a something that is toxic water, and that will cost billions to dispose of. Government is helping Cargill get rid of their hazardous waste products. Cargill is the largest producer of hydrofluorosilicic acid in the world. 250,000 tons of it is dumped in the water just in the U.S. Fluoride inactivates 62 enzymes in the body, inactivates DNA and RNA repair enzymes activity, it is mutagenic, so it causes DNA damage and increases cancers and all other diseases correlated with mutations, disrupts the immune system. If you are iodine deficient fluoride will be used instead of iodine in your thyroid gland because it cannot distinguish between the two. Iodine, bromine, fluoride, and chlorine are all something in chemistry known as halogens. That means they are similar in molecular structure.

The biggest problem is accumulation. Our bodies do not have an efficient mechanism to detoxify fluoride. Any amount of fluoride ever ingested if not excreted initially will stay in the body forever. We can try to mitigate some of the damage, but it is not in any way the effective strategy. Because our body is unable to get rid of the stuff, it is pushed inside calcium-rich tissues like bones. The first sine that you have fluoride toxicity or the first stage of the disease is fragile bones and pain without any medication except painkillers. Dental fluorosis is one visual mark of hypomineralization of tooth enamel caused by ingestion of excessive fluoride. The same thing happens in the bone, and the name of the disease is skeletal fluorosis. The severity of the dental fluorosis is dependent on the dose of fluoride during exposure. In moderate fluorosis, teeth are physically damaged, and it is not just cosmetic concern. The same thing happens in the bones. There is even a gene, a genetic predisposition that causes lactose intolerant people to suck up lead from food. Fluoridated water can free lead and put it in your drinking glass and cooking water. There was a number of published studies that associated higher blood lead levels in children living in communities with artificial water fluoridation. I have discussed lead and that fact that there are no safe levels in the past. Lead is a potent neurotoxin that can lead to developmental delays and other neurological issues. To decrease the hazard of lead exposure in some areas they are treating water supplies with phosphates aimed at inhibiting lead leaching. But what happens if you are African American or Mexican or other lactose intolerant group and then drink fluoridated water with food. Lead from food gets leech out because of the fluoride, or you can just cook with fluoridated water to have the same effect. Effects on the mental state are also a concern.

Anytime you see a pharmaceutical drug that starts with flu that means it is fluoride. For example, Prozac is fluoxetine. Prozac is SSRI drug (Selective serotonin reuptake inhibitors). It takes away anxiety and the pain and makes your mind think that you are not living in the real world. You are put into a state of false reality. Fluoride in death camps did the same thing to prisoners. There are also so far 24 IQ studies that showed correlation beaten very moderate use of fluoride and substantial lowering of the IQ (Effect of fluoridated water on intelligence in 10-12-year-old school children doi: 10.4103/2231-0762.197204). In one Chinese study, they calculated that for each increase of 1 mg/L urinary fluoride there would be a lowering of IQ by 0.59 points. All mention of fluoride impact on the central nervous system in America is ignored, stopped or opposed. It does not just tap water that is contaminated but almost anything with fluid in it like milk, soda, salad dressing, ketchup, baby formula, even solid food for example like cereals. When you water plants in the garden with tap water, they take it up from the ground. You cannot boil it away, and it is very hard to filter out. There is no safe amount for fluoride, it is toxic at any amount, and most of us are already overexposed thru dental products.

After reading little about history and the way companies no matter if they are food, or drug or something third conduct business, you should understand that these companies and people that run them do not care about you. They care about marketing their products to you, but not about you. They will do anything that they can if they can get away with to make their agenda to make money including involvement in war crimes, genocide, torture, exploitation, global scale destruction of any sort. War is one of the biggest business out there. For you to believe that medical practitioners or any other salesmen of any sort are telling you the truth and have caring feelings about you is just propaganda and emotional manipulation designed to promote their agenda by fooling you. When you enter the supermarket, everything there is put on the shelf to make money. There is not one single item in the supermarket that is there to promote health or anything else except to make money to the company that made it. And actually, it is not even companies fault for the grim situation that we have. It is your fault. This is haw, in reality, food market and sales work. Because you do not have control over your basic instincts and your brain is an evolutionary condition the way it is what happens when some food company makes a good healthy product is this. This product does not have any salt, or added sugar or added fat and is full of fiber and so on. If there is no other choice, you will purchase that and eat that. It will be ok; it will not be salty or tasty, but you will manage. However, then some other food company will get the idea to add something to it and will say you know that thing that people purchase why do not we add a little sugar to it to make it taste better. And guess what, you as an impulsive consumer will like it more and then the cycle begins. There will be the third company that will add as much sugar you can tolerate and will add as much fat and artificial tastes and colors and will remove all the fiber and your brain will have dopamine overreaction because this combination of fat and sugar do not exist in nature and you are going to love it. And any other company that will do any other business except making thing full of fat and sugar and salt will go bankrupt. Even when fat is removed from a processed meal, for example, sugar is often added to help disguise the blander taste.

When we say, that process food is bad that is exactly what process means. It means that something is removed. Usually fiber and something is added, usually fat, sugar, salt, and MSG. There is no difference between mac and cheese or pizza or ice cream or chips. When processing removes fiber from flour remaining starch is so easily digested by the human digestive system that there is no difference if we just ate plain crystal sugar. Our body is so well adapted for digestion of amylopectin-a (starch found in wheat) that it is remarkable. So what we have in mac and cheese is sugar from refined flour and saturated fat from cheese, so fat and sugar, combination to get us high. What we have in ice-cream is saturated fat from milk and table sugar, so again fat and sugar. What we have in chips is starch from potato and fat from deep frying and salt and MSG (monosodium glutamate). There is no difference for our brain because what we seek is fat and sugar in the same meal in different combinations, but chemically it is the same meal. Chips can be baked but If you love eating them and tend to eat the whole bag unless someone else gets there first, count on them being fried. If they are baked, the bag will say so and they will cost more and will not taste as good because there will be no dopamine response in the reward mechanism in the brain or not at the scale we would like. It is the same meal again for example when you eat bacon and eggs and bread. It is sugar from bread and fat. Try to eat bacon and eggs without the bread. If you overdo it, you might feel sick from all the fat or why don't you just go and try to eat lard with nothing else. The reason for fiber removal in processed food is that it does not taste good. Fiber does not have a taste what so ever. It is just that we do not like the texture and because there are no calories in it, our brain instinctively detects it as something not worth our time eating. That is the reason we would peel the potato before boiling for example. We do not like the funky texture of the skin. So industry does that to increase texture and color of processed food.

However, what that does is increase the absorption and insulin response. It gets digested rapidly, and when blood sugar drops, we need to eat again, and then we overeat especially because there is added refined sugar and fat. Then obesity comes knocking and then diabetes comes and then because there is no antioxidants in the food or any other phytochemicals to lover inflammation level and all of the toxic overload at the same time we have chronic low-level inflammation. Then that causes cancer and other types of immune diseases. And because we eat too many meat and animal products that are filled with cholesterol and also with no fiber in them as a food for probiotic bacteria we get bad bacteria colony in our gut that feeds on meat or in other words bad microbiome that increases inflammation further and creates whole range of other problems and all of that is because we want our food to taste good. And industry provides. And why industry removes antioxidants and phytochemicals. They do not but what they need to do by law is to pasteurize everything. So when you want to drink for example "healthy" 100 percent no sugar added fruit juice you get sugar and water with fruit flavor with no phytochemical antioxidant what so ever. These phytochemicals are not stable during thermal processing. When the industry starts to boil your juice to kill every potential bacteria and start to add preservatives to it, there are no bacteria anymore, and shelf life is dramatically longer. However, there is nothing in it that is not heat stable any more also including antioxidants. Vitamin C is not stable during thermal processing as well. When you see vitamin C on the box of juice, it is added synthetic vitamin c (ascorbic acid) just to fool you. Also, there is no fiber in the juice as well, so you get nothing different than just sweet water like any regular soft drink like Coke. You need to eat the whole raw fruit to have any health benefit.

Besides all of already mention negative effects, there is still one more negative side of process food, and that is nutrient insufficiency. There is something called macronutrients, and there is something called micronutrients. Macronutrients are sugar, fat, and protein and they contain calories. However, micronutrients are also important for the existence of life although they do not contain any calories. Micronutrients are vitamins, minerals, and antioxidants. The problem is that refined sugar and fat do not have any. It the vegetable oil is "virgin" it might still have some amount of fat soluble vitamins like vitamin E and maybe some small amount of other phytochemicals. However, regular refined oil has zero of everything. It is something called empty calorie, meaning there are zero micronutrients on one calorie. Eating a bag of chips will give you a lot of calories but nothing else. Actually, it is worse than nothing. You will get a lot of salt and excitotoxicity from MSG, and a load of rancid fat and acrylamide. Nutrient deficiency is so pronounced in western diets that in some cases causes serious diseases with a low rate of detection. People who have symptoms of lacking some of the nutrients usually don't know what are they lacking and don't even know that they are deficient at the first place. They think that because they eat so much of the food that they have all minerals and antioxidants and vitamins they need, but in reality, the situation is terrible. Even a healthy diet may lack adequate minerals due to soil depletion and use of synthetic fertilizers. For example, omega three fatty acids, vitamin D, chromium, iodine, and molybdenum were identified as consistently low in more than 90 percent of diet plans. RDA is already artificially lowered to the extreme for some nutrients like vitamin D and iodine. 8 out of 10 people have vitamin E deficiency. Almost half of the US population (48%) consume less than the required amount of magnesium and same applies to vitamin A and vitamin C. When we look into all of the other non-essential trace minerals that we don't understand all of their biochemical actions and don't have RDA for, situation is about 90 to 97 percent deficiency.

As early as 1936, Congress was recognized that the land is lacking micronutrients causing over 99% of the American people to be deficient in some of the essential and trace minerals. Fruit and vegetables today have far fewer nutrients than they did 50 years ago. Potatoes, for example, had lost 100% of vitamin A content, 57% of vitamin C and iron, and 28% of calcium. This data is from the US Department of Agriculture concerning vegetable quality. Over the entire 20th century the average mineral content in cabbage, lettuce, spinach, and tomatoes, declined from 400 mg to less than 50 mg. Mineral depleted soil grows mineral depleted foods. The animals that we eat are being fed these micronutrients depleted vegetables, corn and wheat too. This would translate into the meat that you buy to be also far lower in the level of micronutrients than ever before. Reaching the recommended daily intake of all of the essential and trace micronutrients is difficult, if not impossible, especially for the trace ones, even when following today's most popular diet programs, designed by physicians and nutritionists. We will have to eat whole food vegan, organically grown, nutrient dense diet designed and monitored by professional in order to get all nutrients we need from food. Now imagine what happens when you on top of all of this eat nutrient deprived full of sugar and fat process food made by the food industry. When your main source of antioxidants is coffee, you know that you have a serious problem. Antioxidant levels in foods are measured by a test called ORAC (Oxygen Radical Absorbance Capacity). The higher the ORAC, the higher the antioxidant activity. Antioxidants play a crucial role in your health by lowering free radical damage and neutralizing different toxins and lowering inflammation. Usual antioxidant intake in the US diet is between 3,000 to 5,000 ORAC units per day. It is almost unbelievable how bad American diet is. 40,000-50,000 units a day may be needed to have a measurable effect on antioxidant levels and provide adequate protection from all sources of free radical damage. One hundred grams of raw cocoa powder have for example around 95,500 units, but some part of that is lost during heating when processing it into cocoa powder you find in stores. When you ask big brother The United States Department of Agriculture, previously a publisher of ORAC data what is a response? In 2012 USDA's Nutrient Data Laboratory (NDL) removed the USDA ORAC Database for Selected Foods from the NDL website due to "mounting evidence" that the values indicating antioxidant capacity have no relevance to the effects of specific bioactive compounds, including polyphenols on human health.

Do not worry about it. Just go and eat lard. USDA probably have no "mounting evidence" that sugar and fat in different processed food products are bad either. That is why in recent years industry has tried to do some strange experiments like trying to add blueberry extract into the meat. And when we look into all studies done on antioxidants, there are tens of thousands literary tens of thousands double blind placebo controlled clinical trials so far. We can just look into curcumin studies for example (yellow antioxidant pigment from turmeric powder) and we can see that it kills cancer cells better than leading chemotherapy drugs with no side effect except longevity. Because curcumin and other phytochemicals are hard to absorb USDA will use this as an excuse why phytochemicals don't do anything and why they removed recommendations for ORAC requirement in the diet. However, they do absorb just not in 100 percent manner and for example adding just a pinch of black pepper into the turmeric to create a mix will increase curcumin absorption from turmeric tenfold and you do not even need to buy curcumin supplement especially because there are other antioxidants in turmeric as well. For example, beta-carotene is a pigment, antioxidant, just another phytochemical and need some sort of fat to get absorbed but that does not mean it is not absorbed completely because it will mean that all vegans would be dead from vitamin A deficiency (your body makes it from beta-carotene). However, again industry and government have the interest to fool you. They find some excuses and do studies and everything else they can use. This just shows how corrupted the US Government in reality is, and what length will they go to confuse and abuse their own citizens for the industry interest. I will write about fiber, minerals, phytochemicals, antioxidants and nutrient density in later chapters in more detail and I will cite all the studies.

So how much fat and sugar are there in real life. It is determined that the typical individual in the U.S. eats around 19.5 teaspoons, or 82 grams (g) of sugar, per day. You should eat no more than zero except for sugar found in whole fruits. Fruits contain natural sugars in combination with fiber and antioxidants, and that is less harmful than the sugar found in processed food. Added sugar or "free sugars" refers to any glucose, fructose, and sucrose added to foods and drinks, not just table sugar in crystal form. The phrase does not refer to the regular sugars found in fresh fruit or vegetables because there is no evidence linking these sugars to health problems. They come with fiber, so there is no blood sugar spike, and also they come with antioxidants, so there is no inflammation spike. Why would eating sugar create an inflammation spike?

Burning glucose for energy is not 100% clean reaction. Animals are users. Any animal that is in existence does not create their own energy. Instead, animals get their energy from eating producers that create energy. In other words, animals eat organisms that store sun energy (plants) or eat other consumers. All we eat is just solar energy in different material forms. The purpose of eating is to get glucose. Glucose is the main molecule our bodies use to make energy, and we cannot survive without it. There is a chemical reaction in our bodies called cellular respiration where cells use glucose and oxygen that we breathe from the air to make energy with the creation of byproduct of carbon dioxide, that will be removed from the body and water. The problem is that there is more than just carbon dioxide that is formed. Regular cellular respiration has the electron transport chain in the mitochondria. It is normal conditions that can lead to the formation of reactive oxygen species and cellular damage. In other words, some electrons can escape the electron transport chain and combine with oxygen to form a volatile form of oxygen called a superoxide radical ($O_2^{\bullet-}$). It is one of the reactive oxygen species (ROS) type of free radical. In other words, the process of burning energy that gives us life also gives us death and aging by free radical damage. Naturally, in food, there are some antioxidants to fight free radicals, but when we eat refined sugar, we will have a higher level of inflammation than normal and premature aging. Any sugar that is concentrated is no good even natural ones because of too many empty calories.

Sugars that occur naturally in honey, syrups and fruit juice are even worse. Why? Because there are still refined and usually in the form of fructose (fruit sugar) not in the form of glucose (type our body use). One hundred percent of calories from fructose or any other sugar in that manner that are not in the form of glucose is directly going to the liver to be altered into the glucose. Glucose is the only sugar that our cell use to make energy and also in most animal cells as well. A very similar pathway also operates in plants, fungi, and many bacteria. Other molecules, such as fatty acids and proteins, can also serve as energy sources but only when they are funneled through appropriate enzymatic pathways. So when fructose goes to the liver for the process of chemically altering it will not be a problem except for one thing. The process of altering fructose to glucose is biochemically exactly the same as the process of metabolizing alcohol. One hundred percent the same, and 100 percent the same strain to the liver as alcohol. Alcohol is created by fermentation of fruit or fructose in it actually. In the liver, half of the fructose is converted to glucose, 25 percent to lactate, 15 percent to glycogen and 3 to 5 percent to triglycerides. One byproduct is also bed cholesterol besides triglycerides. When we eat fruit, it does not matter because no matter how much fruit we eat the digestion would be gradual and strain to the liver normal and there is a lot of antioxidants there to fight inflammation. We have been eating fruit for 60 million years. However, when we refined and extract fructose, then it is a different story. It goes directly to the bloodstream and directly to the liver and can cause damage if we overeat. It is the same thing with the alcohol. One glass of wine is fine, but one bottle of vodka is not. If vodka is 35%–95% (usually 40%, minimum) alcohol one lite of it or one bottle will be 400 grams of alcohol. And if 1 gram of fructose is the same as 1 gram of alcohol, then the problem can accrue because we can easily eat a bunch of sugar, but we cannot easily consume one liter of vodka. We can theoretically eat 400 grams of fructose in one sitting, and it would be the same strain to the liver as a one liter of vodka, you just won't feel it in the brain.

For example, sodas are full of sugars, with different types ranging, on average, between 37 grams and 45 grams per 12 ounces serving (equivalent in alcohol content to 80ml of vodka if HFCS (high fructose corn syrup) 65 is used as the sweetener). In recent years, various soda companies have released 'throwback' sodas containing cane sugar instead of HFCS, which is more expensive to them, but almost any soda you buy from a vending machine or at a restaurant is full of HFCS. HFCS 65 is for example used in soft drinks dispensed by Coca-Cola Freestyle machines. HFCS can contribute to a leaky gut syndrome, raise bad cholesterol levels, put unnecessary strain on the liver already bombarded with toxic overload and that can create non-alcoholic fatty liver disease and contributes to fat storage in an entire body, not just in liver creating weight gain. It may also increase your risk of developing cancer. If parents would not like for their children to drink vodka, then they should not let their children drinking Coke either or any other fructose added drinks or food. Also, people that already have issues with the liver in any shape or form not just alcoholics or fatty liver disease sufferers should avoid fructose. And don't get fooled high fructose content is not just in corn syrup. For example, "healthy" agave nectar is high fructose syrup too. The reason that agave nectar does not spike blood sugar much is that all of that fructose need to go to the liver first. This is why high fructose sweeteners are often marketed as "healthy" or "diabetic friendly." The mice getting agave nectar gained less weight and had lower blood sugar and insulin levels in studies. That being said although fructose does not raise blood sugar levels in the short-term, it can contribute to insulin resistance when consumed in large amounts and worsen the condition in long-term but when you do not understand the metabolism of sugars you are an easy target. People with diabetes do not drink alcohol and fructose, in the long run, is bad as much as alcohol is. It can cause major increases in long-term blood sugar and insulin levels, strongly raising the risk of metabolic syndrome and type 2 diabetes. This "healthy" sweetener is even worse than regular sugar. Almost every sugar out there is some sort of combination of sugars when digested. Honey, for example, is fructose (38.2%) and glucose (31%); and disaccharides (~9%) sucrose, maltose, isomaltose, maltulose, turanose, and kojibiose and 20 percent water. Unlike table sugar, it has some trace amounts of enzymes, minerals, vitamins and antioxidant at about 0,5 percent of weight.

Difference between honey and table white sugar is 0,5 percent. Table sugar or sucrose is obtained from sugar cane sugar beets a contains 50 percent glucose and 50 percent fructose. Every fructose molecule in sucrose [table sugar] is bound to a corresponding glucose molecule and must go through an extra metabolic step before it can be utilized, unlike HFCS fructose that is immediately available for fat conversion, whereas sucrose needs a further breakdown. HFCS can be 55 percent fructose and 42 percent glucose (primarily found in sweetened beverages) or 42 percent fructose and 58 percent glucose (used as an ingredient in other packaged foods). Agave nectar has ranged from 56 to 90 percent fructose with the remainder primarily glucose making it one of the highest fructose levels among sweeteners and no nutritional value, all vitamins and minerals are stripped out during the refining process. This is a bad sugar, indeed. Maple syrup is extracted the thick sap of the maple tree, collected from a tap bored into the truck, then boiled to evaporate the excess water. Although low in free fructose, sucrose content was found to range from 51.7 to 75.6% (which is half fructose); glucose and free fructose contents ranged from 0.00 to 9.59%.

The main element that sets maple syrup above refined sugar is the fact that it also contains some minerals and antioxidants. 100 grams of maple syrup contain calcium: 7% of the RDA, potassium: 6% of the RDA, iron: 7% of the RDA, zinc: 28% of the RDA, manganese: 165% of the RDA and at least 24 different antioxidants that would or would not survive the boiling process but keep in mind that it also contains a whole bunch of sugar, so the nutrient density is bad as it gets. It is slightly "less bad" than sugar. Replacing refined sugar with pure, quality maple syrup is likely to yield a net health benefit, but adding it to your diet will just make things worse. 100 grams of molasses in contrast contain calcium: 20% of the RDI, potassium: 42% of the RDI, iron: 26% of the RDI, manganese: 77% of the RDI, magnesium: 61% of the RDA, copper: 24% of the RDI, selenium: 25% of the RDI, vitamin B6: 34% of the RDI and 290 calories instead of 400 for regular table sugar so you would probably need to use more to get the same sweetening effect. Molasses contains several important nutrients and is fairly high in minerals. However, it is also very high in sugar and nutrition density is still low. Molasses is black because of minerals, the darker the color, the more minerals in it. Molasses is derived from refining sugarcane into sugar just like table sugar (it is sucralose in composition, equal parts fructose/glucose) and the only difference is that it was not refined from all of the minerals to create a nice white crystal structure. Molasses varies by the amount of sugar, but it is definitely a better choice than regular white table sugar (if you do not mind your nice white wedding cake becoming brown). Coconut sugar belongs in the same boat as most sugar alternatives. It is healthier than refined sugar but definitely worse than no sugar at all. The main ingredient of coconut sugar is sucrose (70-79%), followed by glucose (3-9%). Sucrose (table sugar) that is made up of half fructose when calculated makes coconut sugar 38-48.5% fructose, which is about the same as table sugar.

Maybe the best option, if you want to avoid fructose (if you have a liver disease for example), is barley malt syrup. Malting grains develops the enzymes required for modifying the grain's starches into various types of sugar, so the sugar is just glucose derived from the grains carbohydrates by digesting them to simple sugars. The composition of barley malt syrup is made of approximately 60% maltose with the rest being made up of glucose and traces of fructose and sucrose. Maltose is just two units of glucose joined. No fruit and vegetables are used, so no fructose what so ever. Malted grain is used to make beer, whiskey, malted milkshakes, malt vinegar and some baked goods, such as malt loaf, bagels, and rich tea biscuits. Sugar obtained from malted barley is still just sugar. It has a moderately higher glycemic index of 40. It is the same as the sucanat. It is a healthier choice to white sugar (GI = 80) or high fructose corn syrup (GI = 87), it is still just sugar. Among all types of sugar tested, this study (Total antioxidant content of alternatives to refined sugar. doi: 10.1016/j.jada.2008.10.014.) found that only blackstrap molasses surpassed malted barley in antioxidant activity. Date sugar scored very close to molasses (but with much fewer calories and a lot of fiber). Blackstrap and dark molasses ranked the highest in terms of antioxidant capacity, followed by date sugar and barley malt syrup. Refined agave nectar, regular sugar, and corn syrup contained minimal antioxidant activity (<0.01 mmol FRAP/100 g); raw cane sugar had a higher FRAP (0.1 mmol/100 g). Dark and blackstrap molasses had the highest FRAP (4.6 to 4.9 mmol/100 g), while maple syrup, brown sugar, and honey showed intermediate antioxidant capacity (0.2 to 0.7 mmol FRAP/100 g). Based on an average intake of refined sugars and the antioxidant activity measured in typical diets, substituting alternative sweeteners could increase antioxidant intake an average of 2.6 mmol/day, similar to the amount found in a serving of berries or nuts. And if you go with blackstrap molasses, your increase will be 4,46 mmol/day for 90 grams of molasses consumed. And you will get some of the minerals too. The problem with substituting alternative sweeteners could be individual taste preferences as well as the level of sweetness. Malt syrup, for example, has that problem. Maltose is not as sweet as other types of sugar, so you will use more sugar and more calories for the same sweetening level. It is only about 30 to 50 % as sweet as sucrose (table sugar) and significantly less sweet than honey (which have fructose in it). The sweetest sugar of them all is fructose so industry naturally likes to use it because it can use less of it for the same effect.

Food formulators widely embraced HFCS, and its use started to grow between the mid-1970s and reached the peak in mid-1990s, mainly as a replacement for sucrose. So why does the industry even use HFCS? The only reason is that it is cheap. And why is it cheap? Because there is a lot of genetically modified corn grown in the US. HFCS has many other advantages compared to sucrose that makes it attractive to food manufacturers that include its sweetness, solubility, and acidity. The High Fructose Corn Syrup Production today is enormous, but industry expanded only slightly over the past five to ten years as it encountered multiple problems. As health-conscious consumers have read the books like these and started to understand little about nutrition they moved away from sodas toward fresh and unprocessed foods and sugar in general. Industry experienced decreased demand and had subsequently lowered annual production. According to data from the US Department of Agriculture (USDA), 90.0% of the HFCS-55 produced today in the United States is sold to beverage manufacturing industries. As HFCS has increasingly been labeled as unhealthy, many soda manufacturers have shifted away from HFCS in favor of traditional sugar. In 2017, both Pepsi and Coca-Cola released versions of their flagship beverages that touted being sweetened with traditional sugar. Nevertheless, HFCS is still considered a low-cost substitute for sugar, maintaining its ubiquitous presence in US sodas and confectionery goods and will be for foreseeable future unless all of the people start to read books about nutrition and educate themselves outside the mainstream media. In the end, HFCS production industry is expected to grow over the next five years. Marketing efforts they can use will have an effect and will work to negate the stigma that HFCS is less healthy than traditional sugar.

One of the strategies applied is to use HFCS-42 and HFCS-55 or in other words industry lowered its fructose content. HCFS-42 is composed of 42 percent fructose, with the remaining sugars being primarily glucose and higher sugars that made the syrup the same as table sugar in terms of fructose level so now there is no difference. Just use a cheaper product. The only problem here is that glucose is not as sweet as fructose so when your lower the fructose content you need to use more of the sugar as a whole to reach the same sweetness level. The net effect is almost the same if you use less of high fructose content syrup or lower lever fructose content syrup except that now you can market the product as something that is as "healthy" as regular table sugar. Operators also benefit from governmental corn subsidies, enabling operators to access low-cost corn in bulk. Because of government interventions like corn subsidies, the low cost of HFCS will be an essential factor that will force the use of HFCS in all products that are marketed to a general population that is not health-conscious. Working out how much sugar, in general, is in your food or drink can be confusing, as it appears in many different forms, not just as added HFCS such as already mention sucrose, glucose, fructose, honey, and others and if you don't know that that is actually sugar you can be fooled. Food producers are not obligated by law to separate added sugars from naturally occurring sugars on a nutrition label, one more tactic to fool you so you will have to be smart. You can find out how much total sugar is in a product by looking for the 'carbohydrates (of which sugars)' figure.

So how much sugar is actually in there? Food manufacturers often put health claims on the front of food labels to fool you into thinking that product is actually healthy. They can legally do this. This can make some foods seem like a healthy choice, when in fact they are full of added sugar. If they remove fat from some product, they will not be able to sell it because it will taste horrible. So what will they do if there is health concern for some food product that became widespread knowledge, like for example saturated fat in milk? They will remove that fat and will label it as "healthy," "low-fat," "diet" or "light." However, they will often have to add more calories in sugar to make them taste good. The really "nice" food companies that care about you will add artificial sweeteners instead of sugar and market that product as healthy low-calorie diet alternative, but you will have to pay more, and most of the time people will just buy sugar added one. The industry also adds large amounts of sugar to foods that are generally not sweet so that they can sell that to the general public that is not health conscious. Examples include yogurt, spaghetti sauce, and breakfast cereals. Breakfast cereals, especially the ones marketed for children, have a high level of added sugar because children will eat more. Some can have as much as 12 grams or 3 teaspoons of sugar in a small 30-gram (1-ounce) serving. These cereals are still far worse than the ones they market to adults. They have 56 percent more sugar, half as much fiber, and 50 percent more sodium. Children usually complain if they are forced to eat unsweetened variety's and industry provides. Some yogurts can contain as much as six teaspoons (29 grams) of sugar in a single container. One cup (245 grams) of low-fat yogurt have around 47 grams of sugar. That is 12 teaspoons. 40% of BBQ sauce is pure sugar. One tablespoon of ketchup contains one teaspoon of sugar. A regular 20-oz (570 ml) bottle of a sports drink will contain eight teaspoons of sugar. Sports drinks are just "sugary drinks." It is same as regular soda and fruit juice. They have also been linked to obesity and metabolic disease. The name is just "sports" drink. Even whole-grain breakfast bars that supposedly are healthy can contain as much as four teaspoons (16 grams) of sugar in one bar. They do not list how much of the sugar in a product is added sugar and how much is natural sugar. They combine all the sugar together and list it as a single amount. Granola is often sold as a low-fat health food. One hundred grams of granola contains nearly 400 calories and over six teaspoons of sugar. "Health bars," cereal bars are usually just candy bars in disguise. A bottle of regular Vitamin water contains 120 calories and 32 grams of sugar. Coke (one can, 330 ml): 7.25 teaspoons of sugar, Sprite (one can): 7.61 teaspoons of sugar, Red Bull (one can): 5.35 teaspoons of sugar, Snickers bar (57 g): 5.83 teaspoons of sugar, Twix bar (57 g): 5.68 teaspoons of sugar.

The problem is that we like our sugar so what to do? Artificial sweeteners do not have the desired effect on the same level on the brain if they are not excitotoxins. Stevia can make thing sweet but will not have dopamine effect on the brain like sugar and especially sugar fat combination so usually it would not be satisfactory as much as chocolate or ice-cream. It will still have a stimulative effect but only for a short time. The industry needs to combine sugar and fat or to use excitotoxin chemicals to give you full blown satiety dopamine sensation. That is the reason for example why Coca-Cola only use aspartame (which is excitotoxin) in Coke Zero. More about excitotoxins later. Artificial sugars are good for the industry in other ways. They can market the products as low or zero calories, healthy, diet and so on but that is opposite of what happens. The first thing that happens when our brain registers the sensation of sweetness in our mouth is the same thing that happened in millions of years of evolution, and that is to tell you to eat it and like it. The brain does not know that thing in our mouth is diet soda. It thinks it is some sweet fruit and it will boost your appetite and give you desire so that you can eat it fast and while you still can before some tiger comes along. Now there is another mechanism that will tell you to stop eating it before you overeat because if you overeat, you might not be able to run away from the tiger. Every time we eat there is satiety mechanism that will tell us when we had enough. With non-caloric artificial sweeteners, we are disconnected. We have stimulant from the sweetness that goes to our brain but no appetite suppressive effect from calories coming into our system. It will leave us wanting more. And because the stimulus is lower than full-blown fat sugar meal the sensation is only temporary. You might feel good drinking diet soda for example but as soon as you stop and sweet sensation signals stop your brain will detect hunger again. Studies that were done usually have found that sweet taste, whether produced by sugar or artificial sweeteners, enhanced human appetite. This revved up in appetite will have led us to overeat even more then we would have without diet soda and end up gaining weight. There is a well-known fact in the industry that came from several large-scale prospective cohort studies that there is a positive correlation between artificial sweetener use and weight gain. While people often choose "diet" or "light" products to lose weight, research studies suggest that artificial sweeteners may actually contribute to weight gain. The most common explanation that the industry likes to use for this counterintuitive finding is what's called reverse causation. People are not fat because they drink diet soda. They drink diet soda because they are fat. So diet soda had nothing to do with it. It is their overall diet that is bad. And I will agree on that, but as always there is more to it.

The San Antonio Heart Study, for example, examined 3,682 adults over a seven to eight-year period in the 1980s. When matched for initial body mass index (BMI), gender, ethnicity, and diet, drinkers of artificially sweetened beverages consistently had higher BMIs at the follow-up, with dose dependence on the amount of consumption. Adding artificially sweetened beverages just encouraged them to eat more. Similar observations have been reported in studies with children too. In nutrition science, there is a psychological effect known as "overcompensation for expected caloric reduction." If you covertly replace someone's soda for diet one or some candy with non-sugary one without target knowing it, his or her caloric intake drops. But people who knowingly are consuming artificial sweeteners may end up eating more calories because overcompensation that comes along later. One of the studies involved giving people an artificially sweetened cereal for breakfast, but only half were told (Effects of aspartame and sucrose on hunger and energy intake in humans. Physiol Behav. 1990 Jun;47(6):1037-44). If there is a lunchtime, the group that understood they have an artificially sweetened cereal ate significantly more calories overall than those that didn't know. The only one that can lose weight on "light" and "diet" food products are the ones that don't realize that they are drinking or eating them. In the meantime, because they do know they will just eat more of the "light" products and will spend more and more money on it without losing any weight. And this is just the psychological side.

There is a physiological component as well. Animals seek food to satisfy the inherent craving for sweetness, even in the absence of energy need. Lack of complete satisfaction further fuels the food-seeking behavior. Reduction in reward response may contribute to obesity especially because artificial sweeteners do not activate the food reward pathways in the same fashion as natural sweeteners and especially not a combination of sugar and fat that most people are accustomed to. There is one more thing. Going off the sugar completely and eating natural foods with added artificial sweeteners are again problematic because the artificial sweeteners, precisely because they are sweet, encourage sugar craving and sugar dependence. They condition the brain to the level of desired sweetness and eating regular food seams as not satisfactory or even as bitter or sour. Sweet intensity of normal unsweetened food is perceived as lower because repeated exposure trains flavor preference. A strong correlation exists between a person's customary intake of a flavor and his preferred intensity for that flavor. Eating healthy whole food diet with added artificial sweeteners will train the brain to except the same level of intensity in other regular foods and will make you to not want to eat them. This behavior is seen in children and adults to just children are more "vocal" about it. By continuing to consume any sweeteners, with or without calories we are unable to train our flavor preferences away from intensely sweet foods. Using artificial sweeteners will make your entire healthy meal feel as unsweetened. It is hard to condition yourself to the natural food level of sweetness even with all of the over sweet banana hybrids and dried fruits that exist today if you eat sugar or artificial sweeteners on the regular bases. If artificially sweetened beverages really help in what they are marketed to do, we will have studies that support that result. We do not, and exactly the opposite is the case, and the industry knows this. It is just another lie for boosting the sales that make people feel better about themselves. And there is one more bonus. The potential toxicity of artificial sweeteners. Some research has associated artificial sweeteners with a wide range of health conditions such as cancers and DNA damage, hepatotoxicity, migraines, and low birth weight. In the U.S., the three most common primary compounds used as sugar substitutes are saccharin (e.g., Sweet'N Low), aspartame (e.g., Equal and NutraSweet), and sucralose (e.g., Splenda). In many other countries, cyclamate and the herbal sweetener stevia are used extensively. Acesulfame-K sold as sweet one is linked with an acute headache and also links to DNA damage. It is proven to be clastogenic (mutagenic agent) and genotoxic at high doses and has caused thyroid tumors in rats. Cyclamate sold as sugar twin was banned more than 40 years ago because of the link with bladder cancer in mice and testicular atrophy in mice. Still legal in Canada and many other countries. Saccharin, discovered by accident while experimenting with coal tar derivate is linked to nausea, vomiting, diarrhea, cancer in offspring of breastfed animals, low birth weight, bladder cancer in people, hepatotoxicity. Sucralose discovered by accident while experimenting at Queen's College in London while trying to formulate a new pesticide (e.g., Splenda) is linked to diarrhea, thymus shrinkage and cecal enlargements in rats. It is a very strong migraine trigger. Worst of them all and linked to more than 75 diseases like lymphomas and leukemia in rats is Aspartame (NutraSweet). Sugar alcohols like sorbitol and xylitol unlike erythritol are not absorbed, and so they ferment in the colon and draw fluid into it and can have a laxative effect. Ok but there are still people who want to taste something sweet but have diabetes, and for them usually, sugar substitutes are must in the diet.

Until some new studies were done the common belief recently was that non-nutritive substitute sweeteners were healthy sugar substitutes because they provide a sweet taste without calories or glycemic effects so they can be extremely beneficial for people who have diabetes. However, results of some epidemiological research have found that consumption of artificially sweetened food, mainly in diet sodas, is associated with increased risk to develop obesity, metabolic syndrome, and more importantly, type 2 diabetes. The problem was that they were considered just to be chemicals that are metabolically inactive in the gut and that they just go truly out the digestive system without promoting metabolic dysregulation. I already mention that artificially sweetened food interferes with learned responses that contribute to sugar cravings and appetite control, but there is also one more thing important to everyone but especially to people with diabetes that use them the most. Artificial sweeteners do have metabolic effects. In this study for example (Sucralose affects glycemic and hormonal responses to an oral glucose load. doi: 10.2337/dc12-2221.) when they give to the obese individuals the amount of sucralose found in a can of coke zero they will get significantly higher blood sugar spike in response to glucose challenge. How much? Twenty percent more insulin level in the blood showing that sucralose causes insulin resistance. And not just sucralose. In this study (Artificial sweeteners induce glucose intolerance by altering the gut microbiota. doi: 10.1038/nature13793.) they tested saccharin (Sweet'N Low), aspartame (Equal and NutraSweet) and sucralose (Splenda) and found that all of them induce glucose intolerance by disturbing the microbiome. They alter microbes that live in our gut. If you eat artificial sweeteners, they will alter the bacteria that grows in our gut because they are hard to absorb, so they stay in our large intestine and ferment. Acesulfame-K was also tested and correlated with changes in gut bacteria. This is also important not just to people with diabetes but to other diseases that are correlated with a digestive system like inflammatory bowel diseases like ulcerative colitis and Crohn's disease. For example, cyclamate was not metabolized when first time injected, and gut bacteria do not know what to do with it. However, after the ten days, 75% of it will get metabolized by gut bacteria into cyclohexylamine and if you stop eating it those bacteria that metabolize it dies back. Cyclohexylamine is very toxic, and the FDA banned it in 1969 but not in Canada and many other countries. So is there any artificial sweetener that is safe.

Stevia is thought to be not that bad because there was some research initially that showed that it is totally harmless. It was later found that it can affect microbiome in the guts of the rats. It gets fermented into a substance named steviol that is mutagenic and causes DNA damage. Humans have the same gut bacteria that ferment stevia. When we eat stevia mutagenic steviol is created and absorbed into our bloodstream. WHO considers 4mg per kg of body weight of stevia safe so you might get away with one stevia sweetened food item a day. So far the only nontoxic artificial sweetener may be Erythritol (Zsweet). It is found naturally in grapes, pears, and melons but yeast is used in industry to make it. It is absorbed in the intestine without fermentation and does not have a laxative effect. It seems that it does not interact with anything or have any metabolism in the bloodstream and it is excreted unchanged in the urine. It does not correlate with any disease, and it might even be helpful. It might be actually antioxidant that is at the same time also sweet (Erythritol is a sweet antioxidant. doi: 10.1016/j.nut.2009.05.004). Erythritol was shown to be an excellent free radical scavenger (antioxidant) in vivo and may help protect against hyperglycemia-induced vascular damage (diabetes). To be safe if you have diabetes and use artificial sweeteners use Erythritol. So far the science shows that this is the best option. In the cited study it was shown that Erythritol protects the agent's oxidative destruction of the red blood cells. Erythritol chemically in the structure looks very similar to mannitol, a well-known antioxidant. Problem with mannitol and other alcohol derived sweeteners like sorbitol or xylitol are that they are not absorbed, unlike erythritol. Only other sweeteners that are sweet and have antioxidant properties at the same time are fruit. They are sweeteners, but they have nutrition at the same time and are healthy too. The best practice to adopt is that if you have sugar craving just eat the whole fruit. Today we live in a globalized society where most of us can find fresh fruit or frozen fruit a whole year long. And also we can use dried fruit as well. It is taste preference so in some cases where it can be done as if you want to sweeten your coffee for example then use erythritol. Date sugar is the healthiest sweetener today and is not really sugar but whole dried dates pulverized into powder. Dates are by weight 80% sugar but they are not correlated with negative effects on weight gain, blood sugar control and actually improve antioxidant stress levels and Hallawi is better than Medjool (Effects of date (Phoenix dactylifera L., Medjool or Hallawi Variety) consumption by healthy subjects on serum glucose and lipid levels and on serum oxidative status: a pilot study. doi: 10.1021/jf901559a). Molasses are in the second place. But because dates or other dried fruit or natural fruit contains fiber it has a thickening effect. If you do not want to thicken coffee or tea for example, then Erythritol can be a choice.

In food items that cannot be sweet the fat is added, salt and usually MSG (Monosodium glutamate) if taste allows. Anytime there are carbohydrates in the meal of any sort, that are actually just one step away from becoming sugar in your digestive system but are not sweet in the mouth the usual thing for the industry to do is to add salt and fat. Fat is added everywhere even in the items that you might think that there is none. Just one tablespoon of oil has 119 calories. How much fat is in just one slice of pizza? Mozzarella is 20% fat by weight. Cheddar, Red Leicester, Double Gloucester, and other hard cheeses are 35%, and Mascarpone is 44%. Can you keep cheese portions small and weigh them to reduce temptation? If you eat addictive foods such as pizza in a state of hunger, you are going to overeat, and because the fat is so concentrated as an energy source, you will think that portion size is small. How much-added oil will we eat when we use cooking methods like deep frying or baking in the oven or when we make salad dressing? Just to give an example here. Chicken Nuggets are chicken skeletal muscle around 40 to 50%. Rest of it is fat, with some blood vessels and nerves, intestines and skin. McDonald is going to say that they just use chicken breast but what they use is chicken breast plus skin, fat, salt, MSG, and other additives. You will see that they are lying if you just look at the nutrition data. You will see that more than 20% by weight is pure fat and that is in raw state before deep frying. That is why they taste softer, and better than dry grilled chicken breast. Fat is added scientifically. Many people do not understand those food companies have laboratories. That they do their own research. These research studies are never published because it is not their goal to push science but only their share of the market. The research they do publish is for manipulation and marketing purposes. The food companies want to know how is our brain attracted to food and how we respond to different stimulus so that they can make their food attractive and addictive when you eat chips for example. There is actual science behind. The result is scientifically engineered combination of salt, sugar, fat, chemicals designed in such a way that we cannot just eat one. Even if we are full, there is still room for one more crunch. Crunch itself is designed to be addictive. The way it breaks between the teeth, the pressure of the bite force, the sound of the crunch. They want people to always at the end of each product to feel the desire to reach for the next one. When you go inside a food company, you will find top-notch scientists and laboratories. When we look into patents that are approved to the food industry, we will see how big of an apparatus is behind food engineering: chemistry, physics, biology.

The food industry can simulate the taste of anything we want, without being actually real.

The most significant finding in the whole history of the food industry is one particular branch of neurotoxins that are called excitotoxins. These chemicals are so crucial for the industry that today you would not be able to find a product that does not have them in one form or the other. Excitotoxins are not derived from food and are not natural, but they can do a lot of good things for the industry. These chemicals for them are a dream come true. Literally, you can take a bowl of boiling water and sprinkle some of the stuff on top, and you will be having the best meal ever. That is what they call soup. You can put them into disgusting products that not even animals would eat, and you will have the best meal ever. Alternatively, you can just take rancid, rotting waste and put them there and you will not feel any rancidity or bad taste what so ever. That is an exact purpose for what they are used. Before WW2 can foods for example where not that tasty because they will lose some of the taste and also had a mild metallic taste. After soldiers in WW2 discovered that Japanese rations taste better and don't have metallic flavor industry became very interested. Now all of this is bad as it is, allowing someone to fool you and sell you waste as food but there is more to it. Excitotoxins are what the name sad that they are. They excite the nerves. So when you put them into your mouth, your brain goes into a high level of neural activity and thinks that that meal is something out of this world. There are receptors for glutamate on the tongue, and then there is overexcitability of the neurons in the brain that follows. Brain cells became very excited, and they start to fire their impulses very rapidly to no end. The first thing that this does is that it desensitizes brain to regular food so after eating a lot of these chemicals even sugary or salty process food seems plain with no flavor. Another thing is that it kills. It kills neurons. Brain cells became exhausted from all that firing, and after the while, they die. In a petri dish, it takes about one hour for them to die and until that time they look normal. They look perfectly healthy and after some time neurons just suddenly die. These chemicals are highly toxic brain poisons. And you cannot get enough of them.

The first excitotoxin discovered and used was amino acid glutamate. Glutamate is a significant component of a broad variety of proteins. Glutamate is created in the central nervous system from glutamine. Consequently, glutamine it is one of the most abundant amino acids in the human body. Any protein in any food that we eat has it. Under normal circumstances, the adequate level is obtained from the diet that there is no need for any to be synthesized by the body itself. Also in normal condition, there is no glutamate in the bloodstream and in the brain in high amount because the body itself is deciding to synthesize it from glutamine or not. When you take already synthetized glutamate, then it is already too late. Nonetheless, glutamine is formally listed as a non-essential amino acid, because the body can synthesize it. For us, it is normal to eat it. The problem arises when you extract it. Only protein-bound glutamate and glutamine exist in food. There is no free glutamate in any food source. If extracted it gets digested rapidly and then overwhelms the brain that had never been exposed to such a high level of it during evolution. And this is a big problem.

Glutamate is a neurotransmitter: a chemical that nerve cells use to send signals to other cells. It will attach itself to the receptor in the neuron, and that triggers the neuron to send the nerve impulse. It is a chemical that brain cells use to communicate with one another. In membrane of the brain cells, there is pore, a small opening. That pore is closed and opens only in one minuscule period until it closes again. Glutamate controls the opening and closing of that pore. Normally there is very little glutamate outside the cell. Minute amounts in millions of the mole. Our brain goes to a lot of trouble to make sure that the level of this neurotransmitter doesn't rise more than that minuscule amount. Only when the glutamate is needed it get loose from its transport protein and gets attached to its receptor, opens up the pore and calcium pours into the brain cell. It is only open in a millionth of the second, just one time until the pore closes again. Once calcium is in, it starts to trigger different processes that at the end makes the nerve fire the impulse. If there is more than normal amount of glutamate and the pore gets open for too long too much calcium will get in. If that happens, the higher level of calcium will trigger uncontrollable firing of the nerve cell. The problem is that it is not a clean process. A nerve cell is unable to fire indefinitely with no rest. What happens is that this uncontrollable firing creates an inflammatory reaction. It will produce free radicals. Then the free radicals will start to oxidize different components of the brain cell by taking electrons from them, and this will create damage. One part of the cell that gets really damaged by this process is mitochondria. Mitochondria are part of the cell that produces all of the energy of the cell. If mitochondria cannot produce adequate amounts of energy, the cell dies. It activates the gene called p53 which is a suicide gene. If a cell gets too damaged, it will kill itself. That is called apoptosis.

Knowing all of this is it reasonable to add this stuff to your food or food of your children or even worse eating it during pregnancy? What are even worse humans are five times more sensitive to effects of excitotoxins then the mouse. We are 20 times more sensitive then rhesus monkey. Newborn babies are four times more sensitive than adults. If you are pregnant and you eat a lot of food that contains glutamate or other excitotoxins that will be passed through the placenta into the fetus. That will permanently damage the babies brain in the time when the brain is being formed. Why are babies so sensitive to glutamate? It is because the enzyme that normally protects the brain is immature and the blood-brain barrier is not fully formed yet. This excitotoxin can alter the way the brain forms. Lower doses can alter the way the cell operates without killing it. It will make the cell overreact so it can, for example, stimulate the secretion of too many hormones, or it might create memory problems or cloud consciousness depending on the area of the brain that is affected. Glutamate also impairs the ability of the brain cells to absorb glucose and can make the brain hypoglycemic. You can have normal blood sugar in the rest of the body, but the brain will be in a state of hypoglycemia. All animal babies that were exposed to glutamate all have similar characteristic later in life. Keep in mind that humans are five times more sensitive then next in line the mouse. Organ weights were small. It causes atrophy. Animals were all morbidly obese, and it was almost impossible to diet off this type of obesity. As soon as animals saw food, there were start to eat uncontrollably. It alters part of the brain (hypothalamus) that control appetite. If there is any part of the brain that will be most sensitive to the effect of injury, it would be hypothalamus. It is a size of a pea and controls an enormous amount of functions. That is part of the brain that we cannot live without. It controls hormones, appetite, sleep-wake cycle, autonomic nervous system (heart, digestive system and so on...), it is a major part of the limbic system of the brain that deals with emotions, and controls immunity. Even the small amounts of glutamate manage to cause early onset of puberty, loss of growth hormone pulsation, and many of these animals were short. Also abnormal reproductive functions with very small litters and infertility. Animals showed antisocial behavior with uncontrollable aggression, and this lasted the entire lifetime of the animal. Impaired cardiovascular responses with a high level of psychical activity. When you ran the heart speeds up, but in these animals, there were a lot of heart arrhythmias, palpitations, and problems. They will have high triglycerides level and cholesterol. Impaired hypothalamic–pituitary–adrenal axis system. That is part of the brain that controls hormones. This and many other effects that I didn't mention was reproducible in any animal, not just mouse. These are all serious things. People think that if they don't get Chinese restaurant syndrome that they are not sensitive and that they are immune to it. This is not an allergy or sensitivity. It is a neurotoxin. Only relevant factor when dealing with neurotoxins is the level of exposure. The industry doesn't deny all of the neurotoxic effects of glutamate and another excitotoxins. They just try to convince people that the level we eat from food is safe. The only other problem is that this neurotoxin produces its effects in an extended period of time silently. You pay the price later. The truth is that you will not associate your medical condition with it. For example, if you have problems with infertility who will be able to correlate that with something that your mother was eating during pregnancy. Playing with fire is never a good idea. Excitotoxins are a hot subject in the field of neuroscience. You will find them in most of the journals that have anything to do with the brain. Every research that deals with brain diseases like Alzheimer or Parkinson's have to take them into account because they can aggravate most of the symptoms of neurological diseases.

Now why is this stuff still allowed in food? Because we use a very small amount of it. They were studies that showed and this is correct that level of glutamate in the food we eat won't cause any form of negative health effect. The primary reason was that no matter how much we eat it would never get into the brain, and that is what makes it safe. And even if it does, the amount in food would not be able to create serious damage. But there are other conflicting studies as well. What some other studies suggest in other hand is that the headaches caused by MSG intake may be related to its harmful impact on neurons in the brain. Although the brain does not have a pain receptor because of the lack of nociceptors, the increase of intracranial pressure due to cell swelling is well known to cause headaches. In this study, for example (The monosodium glutamate symptom complex: assessment in a double-blind, placebo-controlled, randomized study. J Allergy Clin Immunol. 1997 Jun;99(6 Pt 1):757-62.) the conclusion was that oral challenge with MSG-induced symptoms in alleged sensitive persons. Sixty-one subjects entered the study. On initial challenge, 18 (29.5%) responded to neither MSG nor placebo, 6 (9.8%) to both, 15 (24.6%) to placebo, and 22 (36.1%) to MSG. Almost 40 percent of people are a huge amount, and it would be hard to explain it just as a mistake. Total and average severity of symptoms after ingestion of MSG were greater than respective values after placebo ingestion. Rechallenge revealed an apparent threshold dose for reactivity of 2.5 gm MSG. A headache, muscle tightness, numbness/tingling, general weakness, and flushing occurred more frequently after MSG than placebo ingestion. Why some people react to it, and some others don't and why is it that industry can design studies that have people that do not react to glutamate at all?

It is not because of sensitivity. We are all equally sensitive to it. A direct intravenous dose of 50 mg was able to produce similar symptoms. Science is not that tight as the industry would like people to believe. And why different results. It is because of the blood-brain barrier that can be more damaged in some people and have high permeability. If you have a healthy blood-brain barrier, you will be less affected if at all. You can test people and select the ones that are healthier, and they are going to be less affected. Then you can represent the data as safe for the entire population. But what if you are not? What if you don't have 100 percent intact blood-brain barrier impermeability. Hypoglycemia (low blood sugar) is going to disrupt the barrier impermeability for example. Diabetes will do it too. High fevers will do it. Hypertension is one more thing. Head injury, stroke, brain surgery, heat stroke, certain drugs, infections of a different kind, multiple sclerosis and other brain diseases. Natural aging will do it. You could have a mini-stroke that you don't even know that you had. That will open up the brain to the inflow of normal blood from the bloodstream. If you are for example obese, diabetic and you are using insulin, your doctor will tell you to use aspartame (Nutra Sweet) or other artificial sweeteners instead of sugar, and if you have high blood pressure at the same time from obesity, then you are in good predisposition for brain damage.

One more strategy the industry uses is to hide the name MSG on the label. They will say we don't eat much of it and that is true but what about the levels of glutamate that are not calculated because of tactics for hiding it. You don't have to have MSG to have glutamate. You can have it in that exact form as a free amino acid. It is the same thing. How can your free amino acid in this case glutamate from it protein bound? You can break down the protein in different ways one will be to hydrolyze it. So when you see hydrolyzed vegetable protein on the label, it is not. It is hydrolyzed vegetable protein that is actually free glutamate from vegetable protein or in other word disguised MSG. You don't have to use vegetables to do this. Yeast is for example microorganism and has a high level of proteins in it. You can extract free glutamate from that yeast protein, and then you have something called yeast extract. When you see yeast extract on the label, it is MSG. There will also be some other freed amino acids in there beside glutamate-like glycine. Amino acid glycine will magnify the effect of excitotoxicity (Motor neuron degeneration following glycine-mediated excitotoxicity induces spastic paralysis after spinal cord ischemia/reperfusion injury in rabbit Am J Transl Res. 2017; 9(7): 3411–3421.). There are other names they use like natural flavoring. If you extract glutamate from natural sources and it is in its crystal unbound form, then it is not sodium glutamate just free glutamate crystal or "natural" flavoring. Carrageenan is one more. Carrageenan is terrible stuff. It will produce intense inflammation and excitotoxicity in the same time. If you go to the kitchen and make broth stock. You can put MSG in it. When you add that to food on the label will be broth stock, not MSG.

You will have to know the food industry in great detail if you want to be able to recognize all the tactics and names they use. For the average individual, it is a lot of time and effort, and the industry knows it. You will see food that sad contains no MSG but on the label will be yeast extract and natural flavoring. FDA law was made to allow them to do this. Some other disguise names are autolyzed yeast extract, textured protein, soy protein extract, sodium caseinate. Only if it is 99% pure MSG, then they are obliged to put that on the label. And if the form is not even MSG but free amino acid glutamate, then it is even better for them. Soups, dressings, chips, diet foods are one of the worst foods in regards to excitotoxins. If all of those as mentioned above was not bad enough, there is more. There are glutamate receptors throughout the entire body not just in the brain. There is no protective barrier there. For example, the lungs have them. It is a well-established fact that calcium metabolism plays the crucial role in asthma because most of the features in breading like smooth muscle contraction, mucus secretion and neurotransmission to the brain depends on calcium signaling. Calcium channel blockers are used as medication in asthma patients. The spinal cord has them too. So does the heart. Reproductive organs. In experimental animals there where severe arrhythmias caused by glutamate injection and even cases of sudden cardiac arrest. This effect could happen in humans to especially in cases of magnesium deficiency. Magnesium and calcium are two minerals with opposing actions in the body. Calcium stimulates nerves while magnesium soothes them. Calcium overstimulation with magnesium deficiency is a dangerous situation. Glutamate also produces a high level of inflammation, and in cases of low antioxidants intake can cause permanent damage. There are some new studies that correlated glaucoma with excitotoxicity. Glaucoma is not caused by excessive pressure in the eye or poor blood flow but a special form of particular immune excitotoxicity in the retina itself. It is also associated with tumor growth. Stimulating glutamate receptors in tumors cause rapid invasion of the tumor and spreading and forming of metastasis.

Someone once asked me about liquid amino acids and glutamine that bodybuilders use. Luckily they do not contain glutamate but glutamine. At least what I was able to read from the label. Glutamic acid is glutamine, not glutamate. Most free L-glutamic acid in the brain is derived from local synthesis from L-glutamine. Deamination of glutamine via glutaminase produces glutamate. Our body makes glutamate from glutamine, and our body will not increase conversion with the idea to poison itself. It will make only as much as needed. However, hydrolyzed whey protein might be a different story. There is no glutamate on the label, but again there is glutamate in almost every natural protein so hydrolyzing it would free it from its bond and make it in free glutamate form. However, again this is just my speculation because there is no glutamate on the label so I do not know. Do your own research. If you want to be safe just stick to regular whey protein concentrate. Someone also ones asked me if there is any way to protect yourself. In some studies, one effective way in reducing MSG-induced neuronal injury was taking a high dose of vitamin C before exposure. Also, pretreatment of neurons with a low dose of MSG can make neurons tolerant to subsequent high doses of MSG, but I would not play with that. If you are planning to eat a bunch of Chinese food, then take 500 mg of vitamin C before.

Now let us look into the history of all of this. It all started in Japan. In Japan, they used dried grounded kelp seaweed alongside with the salt as a taste enhancer. No one knew why this seaweed enhances the flavor, but they have used it for hundreds of years. In 1908 Japanese chemist, Ikeda Kikunae, was the first to isolate an ingredient in sea kelp that had a distinctive, almost meat-like taste that was the source of enhancement of taste in kelp. It was glutamate that did the job, and he did a lot of research on how this compound can be artificially synthesized. The invention coming out of Kikunae's lab was a white powdered substance called MSG. When announcements of this new product spread, Kikunae proposed describing the flavor as umami—a term derived from the Japanese word for "tasty." Glutamate is not, in reality, any flavor but just the nerve irritant that the brain detects as a flavor when nerves in tongue get exposed to it. MSG means it is just glutamate bound to sodium so monosodium glutamate. It is similar to the regular table salt sodium chloride but with glutamate instead of the chloride. He was smart enough to realize the potential of glutamate for enhancing the taste of food. To put this new product into the market, he made a partnership with Suzuki Company to create a new company named Ajinomoto which means the essence of taste. By the 1930s, tall and slender glass shakers of Ajinomoto were commonly placed on the dinner table in every house in Japan just like salt or hot sauce. When MSG was found in Japanese rations as a source of superior taste there was conference in 1948. The army invited all major food manufacturers. They told them that they had discovered an incredible substance that enhances the taste of food. By 1957 MSG was in everything and food companies assumed it was safe because it is just an amino acid, the breakdown product of a protein. They believed that because it is just nutrient, it must be safe. However, no one actually done any studies on it. It was being added even to the baby foods.

In 1957 two ophthalmology residents did a research project, and they were studying a rare eye disease, and they fed mice MSG. So in 1957 Lucas and Newhouse, the two ophthalmologists found that MSG entirely destroyed all the nerve cells in the retina of the eye. They published the finding, but no one really notices it until ten years later. In 1968 a neuroscientist came across it and decided to use MSG to kill nerves in the eye so that he can observe the pathways of nerves that go from eye to the brain. Well, he did that but what he also did is killed the nerves in the brain too. It was destroying critical parts of the brain as well. At that time, he realized that this is very serious because MSG was everywhere as a food ingredient.

Naively he thought that all he has to do to is to present the information to the food industry and that they will take this stuff out. However, they did not care. So he went to his congressman, and there was a congressional hearing. He presented the evidence and showed the severity of the lesions produced in the brain by MSG. The industry was there and saw the potential problem for upcoming lawsuits. The industry decided that they will voluntarily remove MSG from baby food. Well not really. For ten more years they continued to add it with a disguised name. Even today they add MSG into the baby food. They just created a new class of food with a different name, toddler food to sidestep these restrictions that they imposed on themselves. There were a lot of industry-funded studies after all of this. The response was made in two directions. One of them was that the amount put in food would not do any harm and other one was that there is blood brain barrier that can protect the human brain even if there are toxic effects of MSG. And yes science is correct in both claims. Partially. The real truth is more complicated.

When you are dealing with neurotoxins, there is no such a thing as safe level. Any amount of it that enters the brain will do damage. There is no safe limit. It is the same with any other neurotoxin. There is no safe limit for mercury or lead. Once it enters the brain, it will do some harm. If the scale of the exposure is small the damage is also small. There is no immediate adverse effect. However, in extended period of time even the small amount of damage starts to build up. The only real question is, does the blood-brain barrier is healthy enough to stop glutamate from entering?

Today U.S. Food and Drug Administration (FDA) will say something in the line that the glutamate in MSG is chemically indistinguishable from the glutamate that is naturally present in food proteins. By now after reading this, you know that that has nothing to do with its toxicity because glutamate in natural food is bound and gradually released without overwhelming the brain. The FDA's Department of Health and Human Services notes on its website: "Our bodies ultimately metabolize both sources of glutamate in the same way. An average adult consumes approximately 13 grams of glutamate each day from the protein in food, while intake of added MSG is estimated at around 0.55 grams per day." And again by now, you know that that has nothing to do with it. This statement is also incorrect. A normal grown-up individual eats approximately 13 grams of L-glutamine each day, not glutamate. Big difference. Naturally, 13 grams of glutamine is slowly digested into glutamate, but when you take the crystal form of the pure glutamate stuff, it goes directly to the brain, alters the chemistry and causes damage in about one hour. The proper comparison will be refined sugar. We can eat 500g of sugar a day in the form of natural foods like fruit and be ok. When we refined the stuff, we can eat 500g of it in one big meal and then there is a possibility to end up in a coma.

If you are pregnant and you eat 1 gram of it in a single meal, it will have an effect on the fetus brain. If you are 200-pound male than 1 g of it probably won't harm you. If you have an excellent blood-brain barrier. And the fetus does not so any amount of MSG in refined form is toxic. The blood-brain barrier is what keeps us alive from it so far. And 0,55 grams is just one more lie. A typical serving of food with added MSG contains about 0,5 grams of MSG. It depends on the products. Some have more, some less. And there are disguised amounts of MSG in names as a hydrolyzed protein of yeast extract that does not calculate into this 0,5 average. Consuming more than 3 grams of MSG in food at one time is unlikely. But again it depends on what you eat and how much. The anecdotal threshold dose that causes symptoms to some people may be around 3 grams in a single meal. So if you eat less of it, you would not have any symptoms. The studies done on Chinese restaurant syndrome don't show in reality much of anything. But that does not mean that MSG will not kill some of the brain cells anyway. And that is a real scientific problem with this silent killer. It does its job like professional. You do not see or feel anything but the end result may be dead brain cells anyway. By saying it is all ok, it is safe and so on government is going to create a situation in which some individuals that like MSG food too much will overeat it thinking that it is fine. In China and Japan, they tend to put multiple spoons of the stuff to the meals. Thinking that MSG is just some Chinese restaurant syndrome chemical that will give you a migraine and nothing else is a misinterpretation of scientific data. What if that individual is a pregnant mother with a fetus that does not have a fully developed blood-brain barrier and protective enzymes. In most of the scenarios, you will not ever notice the adverse effects of MSG directly, but you will notice them in life. Later in life. And you will never correlate the two. So what the final verdict on glutamate? It is safe, and it is neurotoxic at the same time. It depends on the situation. However, the situation here is that glutamate is not the end of it. Glutamate is not the only excitotoxin out there. More chemicals do the same.

One of them that have made the industry so happy is the chemical that does all the things that excitotoxins do but unlike MSG is sweet to the taste. It is chemical known as aspartame (Nutra Sweet). When the industry removes fat from the product, it has to add something to make that product tasty again. So what they do is they add something back to increase the taste, usually sugar. If the product is not sweet, then sugar is no option. Then what they do is they will add MSG and salt. The response in the brain from excitotoxins will compensate for missing sugar. However, then the problem arises. What will you add back if a product needs to be sweet? In that case, they can add other artificial sweeteners, but that will not trigger the brain in the same manner as sugar will so they have a problem. The problem that sweet tasting excitotoxin will solve. Think of aspartame as sweet MSG substitute. In cases when they need to have both sugar and fat removed they can add excitotoxins to have the desired effect. That is why MSG soup is tasty without any calories. That is why diet Coke is tasty without any calories. They will add stimulants to it like caffeine and excitotoxins like aspartame that have a sweet taste and will stimulate the brain in the same time, so the response from the brain will be like you have eaten something that actually contains sugar. Drinking diet sodas can be addictive because of this stimulative effect. When we use a stimulant, we become excited. By reacting with our dopamine system, the stimulant provides us with pleasure and euphoria which motivates us to consume the same stimulant again in order to experience a repeated feeling of reward (a process is identified as positive re-enforcement). Another side of this, known as negative re-enforcement, is sudden discontinuation of addictive stimulants that can result in cravings, which is essentially the feeling of wanting to avoid the discomfort that develops once the artificial high of the stimulant has gone. Within both of these processes, we are left wanting more. In fact, the memory for cocaine addiction resides within the glutamate receptor (Group III metabotropic glutamate receptors and drug addiction doi: 10.1007/s11684-013-0291-1). In response to drug exposure, these receptors in neurons show marked and dynamic changes in expression. Emerging evidence ties them to the remodeling of excitatory synapses and persistent drug seeking. The high level of expression of mGluR7 glutamate receptors in the limbic reward circuitry implies its roles in drug addiction. In fact, evidence associates this receptor with addictive effects of psychostimulants, alcohol, and opiates.

The history of aspartame is one of the interesting ones. Back in 1965 while working on an ulcer drug, James Schlatter, a chemist at G.D. Searle, accidentally discovered aspartame, a substance that is 180 times sweeter than sugar yet has no calories. He was recrystallizing aspartame from ethanol. The compound spilled on the outside of the flask, and some of it stuck on to his fingers. He forgot about it and licked his fingers to pick up a piece of paper and noticed an overpowering sweet taste.

In 1967 Searle begins the safety tests on aspartame that are necessary for applying for FDA approval of food additives. Seven infant monkeys were administered aspartame mixed in milk. One died after 300 days. Five others (out of seven total) had grand mal seizures. The results were withheld from the FDA when G.D. Searle submitted its initial applications. Why did the mix aspartame with milk? Because milk will slow down the digestion of it to some extent in the hope that it would not overwhelm the brain in a short time and cause damage. The bigger problem was that they tried to hide the results. A couple of years later Searle Company executives had created the internal policy memo in which they were describing different psychological tactics the company should use to bring the FDA into a "subconscious spirit of participation" with them on aspartame and get FDA regulators into the "habit of saying, Yes." By that time there were more not industry-funded studies.

Neuroscientist Dr. John Olney (that pioneering research with monosodium glutamate was responsible for having it removed from baby foods) did a couple of them and by that time already informed the Searle Company that his studies showed that aspartic acid (one of the ingredients of aspartame) is causing holes in the brains of infant mice. But by 1973 after spending tens of millions of dollars conducting safety tests, Searle Company applied for FDA approval and submitted 11 pivotal studies and did 113 studies in support of aspartame's safety in following years. One year later the FDA granted aspartame its first approval for restricted use in dry foods. Same year two men Jim Turner and Dr. John Olney filed the first objections against aspartame's approval. Two years later their petition triggered an FDA investigation of the laboratory practices of aspartame's manufacturer, G.D. Searle. The investigation found that Searle's testing procedures were unscientific, full of errors and manipulated data. The researchers report they: "Had never seen anything as bad as Searle's testing." G.D. Searle company in the crusade to get approval conducted the line of studies on animals. When they submitted this to the FDA, there was some question about the studies. One way they tried to manipulate the data was that they showed in the studies that there are no significantly more tumors in the test group than in the control group. When some of the neuroscientists that work for FDA looked at the data, they saw that this is correct, but then there were other problems. Both groups had significantly higher tumor rates than normal average, especially for the brain tumors. This can happen when someone tries to manipulate data and represent some of the control rats with tumors as a part of the control group. This will lower the tumor rate in a test group, it will rise it in control group, and at the end, they can say that it does not cause any tumor or what so ever but then both control group and the test group will have significantly higher tumor rates than normal average.

So they requested research to be done by the Bureau of foods which were the precursor to the FDA. Dr. Jerome Bressler was in charge of the group that looked through the research that had been done by Searl. In his report, he stated that there where misinterpretation of the data and that it was a world worst research. The record notices that 98 of the 196 animals died during one of Searle's studies and weren't autopsied until later dates. Numerous errors and discrepancies are noted. For instance, a rat was recorded alive, then dead, then alive, then dead again. They found that some of the animals that died after aspartame Searl scientist did not autopsy to full year later. After that period the flesh was putrefied, and there was no possible way to do an autopsy. However, they represented that they had done autopsies and that animals are normal. They were cutting tumors out and saying that animals are healthy. They had animal tissue that had obvious tumors in it that were reported normal. Testicular atrophy was not noted. There where an effort to cover up the negative effects to get approval. If they did normal research aspartame would not be approved and they realized that.

The FDA formally requested the U.S. Attorney's office to begin grand jury procedures to review whether charges should be filed toward Searle for deliberately misleading conclusions and "concealing material facts and making false statements" in aspartame safety tests. That was the first time in the FDA's history (which is already corrupt institution to begin with) that they asked for a criminal investigation of a manufacturer. While the grand jury inquiry is undertaken, Sidley & Austin, the law firm representing Searle, had begun the job of negotiations with the U.S. Attorney in charge of the investigation, Samuel Skinner. Samuel Skinner will leave the U.S. Attorney's office later that year and will take a job with Searle's law firm Sidley and Ostin. In the same time, G. D. Searle is going to hire the prominent Washington insider Donald Rumsfeld as the new CEO. A former Member of Congress and Secretary of Defense in the Ford Administration. Yes, that Donald Rumsfeld. Rumsfeld was appointed Secretary of Defense for a second time in January 2001 by President George W. Bush. That medal that Rumsfeld received in 2004 was the Presidential Medal of Freedom. "Freedom" proposes the right to use your influential associates in Washington to support your company's hazardous substance for human consumption and make a fat bonus on the way out the door. It also means you can drop bombs on other countries. It also means you can bribe U.S. Attorney in charge of the investigation. After U.S. Attorney Skinner's withdrawal and resignation, there were significant stalls in the Searle grand jury investigation for so long that the statute of limitations on the aspartame charges had run out. Assistant US attorney William Conlon who was assigned to the grand jury investigation let the statute of limitations to run out. He was hired fifteen months later by the same Searl law firm Sidley & Austin. The grand jury investigation was dropped. Two years later in 1979, the FDA established a Public Board of Inquiry to rule on safety issues surrounding NutraSweet. The Public Board of Inquiry conclusion was that aspartame should not be approved until further research are done. The board stated that: "It has not been presented with proof of reasonable certainty that aspartame is safe for use as a food additive." By 1980 the FDA outlaws aspartame from use after having three autonomous scientific studies of the sweetener. It was concluded that one primary health effects were that it had a high chance of inducing brain tumors. We also need to keep in mind that back in that time there was no requirement for the FDA to examine effects on the brain from food additives. There were never any studies done to examine the effect of aspartame on long-term or even short-term neurological effect.

Cancer studies turned brain tumor, but that are cancer studies, not brain studies. Cancer studies were the primary and the only one that they ever investigated. Despite all of this at this point it was clear that aspartame was not fit to be used in foods and banned stayed in place, but not for long.

In 1981 Ronald Reagan was sworn in as President of the United States. His transition team included Donald Rumsfeld, CEO of G. D. Searle. Rumsfeld appointed Dr. Arthur Hull Hayes Jr. to be the new FDA Commissioner. Even before that one of the first things that Ronald Reagan did when he was sworn in as a president was to suspend the authority of the FDA commissioner to take any actions. There was obviously a fear that Commissioner was going to do something about aspartame before he leaves the office. That will make things more difficult for them so Regan suspended the authority of the FDA commissioner until they can elect a new one in a month or so. In that month the old FDA commissioner was prevented from taking any actions. It did not take long for the new FDA Commissioner handpicked by Donald Rumsfeld, CEO of G. D. Searle to approve the chemical substance that is made by the G. D. Searle. New FDA commissioner selected a 5-person Scientific Commission to evaluate the board of inquiry's decision. It took just a couple of weeks when presented with all of the toxic effects of the substance for the panel to decide 3-2 in favor of supporting the ban of aspartame. Hull then resolved to different tactic. He appointed a 6th member to the board, which created a tie in the voting, 3-3. Then Hull himself decided to break the tie and approve aspartame for use personally. Hull later left the FDA under several allegations, served briefly at New York Medical College as a cover, and then took a position as a consultant (1000$ per day) basically to do nothing with Burston-Marsteller. Burston-Marsteller is the main public relations firm for both Monsanto and GD Searle. Since that time he disappeared and has never spoken publicly about aspartame. Seven of the key people that made decisions in this entire process that made aspartame go through the entire process ended up leaving their jobs and getting a new job for some of the Nutra Sweet using industries. In 1985, Monsanto decided to purchase the aspartame patent from G.D. Searle.

Also beginning in the middle 1980s, the FDA dissuaded and actually prevented the National Toxicology Program from doing any long-term cancer research on aspartame. So what was left is hundreds of industry founded studies that showed nothing, 100% safe rate and over 90 of independently done studies that in more than 90% of them showed increase cancer risk and many other adverse effects. Scientific studies have been carried out with conclusion raging from "safe under all conditions" to "unsafe at any dose."

There is a well-documented increase in incident rates of brain tumors in the year 1985 that remained elevated to this day. National Cancer Institute recorded an impressive increase of primary brain cancer rate since 1985. At that time this trend was singularly attributed to more innovative scanning and diagnostic procedures. The problem is that adequate brain scanning devices were widely available for at least ten years prior to 1985. Also, incidents of another form of cancers outside of the brain remained the same and in some cases declined. Aspartame was fully marketed by 1983. Already by 1984, there were 10% increase of brain cancer rate in U.S. and incidence of brain lymphoma, a type of aggressive brain tumor jumped 60%.

In the gut, aspartame is broken down to release methanol and two amino acids phenylalanine, and aspartate. About 50% of it is aspartic acid, 40% of it is phenylalanine, and 10% of it is wood alcohol or methanol. Methanol is further metabolized into formaldehyde. You might know formaldehyde as embalming fluid. The body cannot get rid of formaldehyde. Any amount of it the body stores. The industry has made a big deal about how there is a methyl group which is found in all fruits and vegetables. Anything that we eat has methyl groups so eating methanol in aspartame is no big deal and concentrations of formaldehyde in comparison is minuscule. The amount of formaldehyde we eat from fruit is much more than the amount we could get from aspartame. You will hear this with any doctor or research that is design to defend the use of aspartame. But again they don't tell the whole truth. When the body metabolizes aspartame, you end up with a small amount of formaldehyde, but that formaldehyde is in free form. When you eat fruit, you take more methanol, but that methanol is bound to pectin. Humans lack the enzyme to break down pectin. We are unable to split methanol from pectin. It goes through the body without doing any damage whatsoever. Even if there is more of the methanol in fruit and vegetables in reality that methanol is irrelevant. In aspartame, the free methanol and then free formaldehyde even in the minute amounts are dangerous because the accumulative toxic effect of it. Beside the methanol, in nature, we are eating the same amount of ethanol in fruit or vegetables. There are methanol and ethanol in fruits, and they counteract each other. When G. D. Searle did experiment with monkeys, aspartame give those monkeys grand mal seizures. Monkeys have a higher reaction to ethanol then humans. Regular alcohol like wine. In other hands, they have really high resistance to methanol. Much higher than humans. Even with high resistance, and even though they were fed aspartame with milk, they still had seizures, and one died from cardiac arrest caused by overstimulation of the nervous system.

Beside methanol aspartic acid is excitotoxin and phenylalanine had been showed to cross the blood-brain barrier, and it is a precursor of norepinephrine (adrenalin in the brain). Phenylalanine occurs naturally in the brain. It is not that bad but if we have an unnaturally high level of it can be very bad. There is a medical disorder that affects 1 in 10,000 people known as PKU (Phenylketonuria). It is an overabundance of Phenylalanine in the brain because the body inability to process it. If you add phenylalanine to someone that does not have PKU you can trigger very bad response. Excess amounts of phenylalanine are linked to a reduction in serotonin production. Phenylalanine can trigger for example manic attack in people who are suffering from manic depression. It is being known for a long time, and there are also studies that when you take aspartame with carbohydrates, you will decrease the availability of l-tryptophan in the brain which is a building block for serotonin. It can also trigger regular depletion in susceptible individuals. In one study (Adverse reactions to aspartame: double-blind challenge in patients from a vulnerable population. Biol Psychiatry. 1993 Jul 1-15;34(1-2):13-7.) they even had to stop the experiment. Although the protocol required the recruitment of 40 patients with unipolar depression and 40 without any psychiatric history, the project was halted by the Institutional Review Board after the total of 13 individuals had completed the study because of the severity of the reactions in a group of subjects with a history of depression. It was concluded that it was unethical to continue the study. In this case also the Nutra Sweet company refused to provide the product for the testing and even refused to sell it to them. Researchers had to find it in the third party vendors. In one of the new studies of the effect of aspartame on mood disorders done back in 2014 (Neurobehavioral effects of aspartame consumption. doi: 10.1002/nur.21595.) they took regular healthy people and put them on high aspartame diet. Healthy adults who consumed a study-prepared high-aspartame diet (25 mg/kg body weight/day) for 8 days and a low-aspartame diet (10 mg/kg body weight/day) for 8 days, with a 2-week washout between the diets, were examined for within-subject differences in cognition, depression, mood, and headache. When consuming high-aspartame diets, participants had a more irritable mood, exhibited more depression, and performed worse on spatial orientation tests. This where all healthy people with no history of mental illness. Now, how much high dose of 25 mg/kg body weight/day in actuality is? Well FDA put the safe upper limit at 50 mg/kg body weight/day. High consumption level examined here was well under the maximum acceptable daily intake level of 40-50 mg. And this is just eight days. Consuming this stuff in prolonged period can have even more severe effects.

You can read all of this now but just several decades ago it was a heresy to talk about the pandemic of obesity and how much exactly process food is bad. And it is a global problem now. A western diet with sugar, white flour, animal products, fat and so on had replaced beans, seeds, nuts, whole grains. Promoting healthy food like beans do not go along well with big business. It is not just big tobacco any more but Big Soda, Big Mac and so on... All of these industries protect themselves by using the same tactics. Some of the tactics include lobbying, lawsuits, industry-funded research, marketing. In 2003, for example, the World Health Organization released a draft report outlining the global strategy to address issues of diet advocating for things that the industry did not like, like cutting down on sugar and fat intake. Within days' food industry enlisted the support the officials high in the U.S. government and led a campaign against both the draft and the WHO itself culminating in the Congress threatened to withdraw U.S. founding of the WHO. For example, the same thing happened before when the U.S. defended the tobacco industry. However, the threat from the sugar industry was considered by WHO insiders as even worse from any other previous pressure they ever got. As reviled in internal memo (Why the Bush administration and the global sugar industry are determined to demolish the 2004 WHO global strategy on a diet, physical activity and health. Public Health Nutr. 2004 May;7(3):369-80) U.S. government had a list of demands like deletion of all references to WHO/FHO expert consultation report, deletion of all references to sugar, fat, salt and oils, deletion or modification of all references on the issue on marketing and advertising to children. The political pressure failed to make the WHO withdraw the report but manage to force the "watering down" many of the recommendations. The article named: "Diet, nutrition and the prevention of chronic disease" was formally launched and concluded that a diet low in saturated fat, sugar and salt and high in fruit and vegetables was required to tackle the epidemic rise of chronic diseases worldwide. So now even the WHO, a globalist institution controlled by special interest are kind of advocating adding more of the vegan diet to the average western lifestyle. However, gone was a reference to the comprehensive scientific report, gone was its call for recommendations to be translated into the national diet guidelines, into so-called food pyramid. From 2003 the same was repeated over and over again. The U.S. is blocking consensus on action on non-communicable diseases.

Processing is not always bad. It can also be used for increasing the nutritional value and profile of the food. It is the only problem that our brain seeks calories, not nutrition and that in nature nutrition comes along with calories. There is no separation. So processing food to make it more palatable is not a good thing in nutrition sense. However, sometimes processing can be used in exactly the opposite way to increase nutrition. One good example of it is cacao powder. The processing of cacao is what it gave it "superfood" status. The cocoa beans naturally have energy stored in the form of saturated fat. The same fat you can find in butter or any other animal products. In this case, what industry does is actually grind then heat and press the beans liquor to remove its fat content out of it. In the first step after collection, the seeds are placed where they can ferment. Then they are dried, and the nibs are then milled to create cocoa liquor (cocoa particles suspended in cocoa butter). There is no such thing as raw cacao because if fermentation is interrupted, the resulting cocoa may be ruined if underdone. The cocoa seed maintains a flavor similar to raw potatoes. Another way is to treat cocoa nibs with alkalization, usually with potassium carbonate, to develop the flavor and color. However, what is important is that the cocoa liquor is pressed to extract the cocoa butter, leaving a solid mass called cocoa press cake. The amount of butter extracted from the liquor is controlled by the manufacturer to produce press cake with different proportions of fat. The cocoa press cake is broken into small pieces to form kibbled press cake, which is then pulverized to form cocoa powder. The cocoa butter is later used in the manufacture of chocolate and with added sugar and powdered milk it cocoa powder loses its good nutrition profile. So "the secret" of cocoa high "superfood" nutrition density is actually the removal of its fat content and not just high nutrition of the cocoa beans itself. When you remove the macronutrient calories and in the same time leave all the micronutrient polyphenols and minerals in the bean, then you are lowering the number of calories (some are still left in the bean in the fat that is not removed), and you are increasing the relative amount of micronutrient content ratio to one calorie. Processing, in this case, has created the opposite effect of regular processing directly when excess fat and sugar is added to increase the taste of the product. You can replicate the same processing at home to increase the nutrition profile of your diet without adding any excess calories. Wholly grail of nutrition science. To increase the level of nutrients and prevent deficiencies without eating more calories and getting fat. Or decreasing the level of calories in the diet to lose weight without suffering from nutrient deficiencies. Now you have learned "the secret" knowledge of nutrient density.

How can you do this at home? You just replicate the same process with some other food products that have the calorie reserve in the form of fat. For example, most of the nuts and seeds have high-fat content. So what can you do? How can you replicate these, you don't have cocoa liquor press-machine? Actually, you can if you want. It is called home oil extraction, and many of the juices have the capability to extract oil at home from seeds with some added parts. These home oil extraction devices are designed for raw oil extraction for a health-oriented people who do not want to use refined rancid fats and want fresh squeeze homemade oil for their salad. If you want for example to use omega three oil, it will get rancid immediately after extraction, as soon as it has contact with oxygen it is gone. Purchasing the flaxseed oil in bottles in the stores is not recommended, and home oil extraction is a much better option if you want omega three oil as a salad dressing. However, now that you have the knowledge of "the secret" you will use these in the opposite direction. You will throw away extracted oil and only eat the pulp in your muesli. If you take 100 grams of sesame seeds for example (raw, if heated they will use some of the phytochemicals that are not thermo-stabile) and put them through oil extraction machine it will extract a big chunk of its oil content. One hundred grams of sesame seed has 48 grams of fat. Half of its weight is fat. The machine generally can extract about 40% by weight varying according to the nature of seeds you will be left with 8 grams of non-extracted fat (just enough to aid absorption of fat-soluble phytochemicals). The amount of calorie extracted will be 360 and number of still remaining calories 205. If you add 30 grams of "raw" cocoa powder and let say 10 grams of ground cinnamon, you will have a mixture that has 298 calories total. For those 300 calories which is about 15% of average grown men daily calorie requirement, we will have (if we used organic products that are grown in mineral-rich soil) 1111mg of calcium which is more than in one liter of milk and 111% RDA, 584% RDA for copper, 244% RDA for iron, 233% RDA for manganese, 121% RDA for magnesium, 122% RDA for phosphorous, 91% RDA for zinc, 71% for selenium, 28,2 grams of fiber for 74% RDA, 24 grams of protein and 41,000 units on ORAC scale. In comparison 2 whole eggs with 2 large slices of whole wheat bread and nothing else will have 353 calories and 18% RDA for calcium, 23% RDA for copper, 40% RDA for iron, 82% RDA for manganese, 17% RDA for magnesium, 48% RDA for phosphorous, 22% RDA for zinc, 22% for selenium, 5,2 grams of fiber for 14% RDA, 21,8 grams of protein and 1160 units on ORAC scale with 328,2mg of cholesterol for 170%RDA (ideally this number will be zero). Keep in mind that both eggs and whole wheat bread are whole foods and that there are people out there that will advocate for the use of eggs and whole wheat bread as a best of the best. What do you think will give you more satiety, 100 grams of sesame pulp, cocoa powder, cinnamon mixture with 28,2 grams of fiber (you will have a hard time eating all of this because fiber gets bloated in the presence of fluid) or 2 eggs with two slices of whole wheat bread (most the people will eat white bread). Both of these meals are made from whole foods that in reality can be a lot of different things. Meat is whole food so is honey.

Not all things are made equal, and we need to use a scientific approach when designing meal plans not just whole food or not just even a whole food vegan label. It is better to eat whole food instead of process food, but this is just for the beginners, for the average couch potato that doesn't understand and don't care about anything. Using techniques like "the secret" and others can give completely different nutrition profile. Sometimes even extraction of fiber can be a positive measure for increasing nutrition profile of your diet. If you process fiber out of vegetables that are full with nutrients but low in calories and full of fiber that limits our capacity for eating them in large amounts, we can process fiber out or in other words extract the fluid from them. Juicing greens have its benefits because there are not many calories in them and the fluid is full of nutrients. If you eat enough fiber in the other meals, you can add this practice for increasing the nutrition content of your diet. If you don't want to change anything about your diet you can use these "secret" techniques just as added bonus couple of times a week. You can eat these type of muesli let say two times a week, and you can juice some of the vegetables two or three times in the week just to protect yourself from deficiencies and to increase antioxidant value of your diet. If you do not want to do anything for your health or lifestyle just do this. It will help you more than any pharmaceutical drug or therapy or supplement, and it is dirt cheap. You just need to spend a couple of hours a week in the kitchen.

Protein

"I got 99 problems, and protein is not one of them "- Vegan proverb.

Maybe one of the most asked question in vegetarian and vegan movement is: where did you get your protein. It is so embedded in the subconscious mind of people through all of the mainstream propaganda and marketing that protein is something essential if not the most important so if anything else we need to consume animal products to get protein. The second question is: ok if you do not eat meat can you get it from milk? Wright, we have to get our protein from somewhere, so if not meat that it must be milk. We will address this about milk in the next chapter. Many people during the year had asked me where did you get your protein, and frankly, I am sick and tired of answering that question. Finally let us have real scientific analysis of protein issue so that you can have an adequate understanding of entire "problem." If you are a vegan yourself, you will know exactly what to say to people when they ask this question, so stick around.

Firstly, in the entire nutrition community protein is excepted as something that is essential no question asked. Real enthusiasm started almost immediately after it was first discovered. It was called the essence of life and so on. In the 1890s the USDA recommended an average of 110g of dietary protein per day for an average man. In the 1950 even UN recognized a something they called "The world protein gap" and that when looking at indigenous people "deficiency of protein in the diet is the most serious and widespread problem in the world." Of course, America in that time had postwar surplus-disposal problem of powdered milk. There was in that time even a disease named Kwashiorkor blamed on protein deficiency. It will be later found that it has nothing to do with protein what so ever. However, when anthropologist studies and fossil record showed that hominins lived on average of 15 to 20 grams of protein a day there was a so-called a "Great protein fiasco" back in the 1970s. Industry and big pharma did not like that. There were massive recalculation and reduction in human protein requirements and so-called "world protein gap" was mention no more. It disappeared like it never existed. For example, an infant protein requirement in 1948 was at 13 percent of daily calories and in 1974 was at 5.4 percent of calories.

However, still, this is not the real numbers and do not add up to the evolution of our species. It was as high as an industry can get away with. To this day there are paleo, keto and so on diet people that are obsessing about protein. If you are like them then the protein is the must. No debate there. All we can talk about really is fat and carbs. So if you need your protein to be "adequate" then what is left is fat and carbohydrates. You can have a high carb diet and low fat or another way around high fat keto low carb diet. So, what is your diet? What is the healthiest? Did you ever hear of low protein diet or high protein diet? Maybe if you are into bodybuilding or have kidney failure. Three macronutrients are protein, fat, and carbohydrates but no nutritional expert will ever tell you the truth about protein. They are not paid to do so. They will talk about everything they can except a real amount of protein your body needs. Everybody talks about fats and carbs, but suspiciously enough nobody ever talks about protein. The only thing you will hear it is essential for life, building blocks of every cell on earth and you need the most you can get because the more you get it, the better. Typical American can eat on a regular basis more than 90 grams of protein a day (Current protein intake in America: analysis of the National Health and Nutrition Examination Survey, 2003–2004 doi.org/10.1093/ajcn/87.5.1554S). Bodybuilders do to the marketing will end up eating up to 200 grams of protein a day. That is not health promoting by any standard, but that is not what industry say to these people. They say the more, the better. The more protein, the faster the muscle will grow. That is by the way, another lie. And why the industry does that? Well, first so that you will overeat on "high quality" protein because your body needs it so your diet will be focused on meat and dairy. However, the second reason is whey. It was a waste product that industry dumped down the sewage until someone got the idea to sell it to the bodybuilders. They dehydrated the whey and what was left was bacteria filled with protein. Now you will pay a lot of money to get that bacteria powder so that you will have more protein in the diet. Something you do not need. It is all a scam. Every single thing, and by reading this chapter to the end you will understand why.

Why don't we first look around the world and see where the protein is? In nature we were tropical creatures so where is the protein if we look to our ancestor's species and indigenous people of today. Let us look our real ancestors, meaning indigenous hominins in warm climates where we evolve and let us look where and how much protein they had in their diets. They did not have a diet that was focused on protein, only Neanderthals in the Far North did. However, for us, it is a completely different story. Before the technology allowed humans to go above 40 parallel what do you think how much protein did we eat on a regular basis? It was around 15 to 20 grams daily. All of the science showed us repeatedly and conclusively with no doubts that if you eat less protein, you will be healthier and if you eat whole food plant-based diet you will be the most healthier and you will live longer. That is what science has repeatedly shown us through the experiments. When you eat plant-based, you get less, and you get a less complete protein. Avoiding complete protein is the one reason that was shown with extensive research that is the main culprit in longevity and health. Eating much less protein then the standard American diet eaters do. And if you do don't want to believe keep reading. When you avoid excessive food intake and eat mostly starch or other plant-based products, what is the side effect of that? The side effects are that simply you eat much less complete protein, and that is the secret industry knows but don't want to tell you. Science is here and had been here for a long period of time. When all of those scientist went to the blue zones of longevity to research indigenous people and to find the reason why are they so long living and healthy, they could just tell you the truth. They eat much less protein. But they did not. And why? Why is it so hard for the Western Civilization to accept that protein is poison in excessive amounts? Because you will have to eat less pizza? If you eat less amounts of animal products, you will automatically eat less protein. For the reason that you will understand by the end of this chapter, protein have become the "Holy Cow" of nutrition, and not by accident.

It is politically, scientifically, socially and in any other way forbidden to talk the real truth about protein. Just look at the nutritional experts and medical doctors of today. For them it is just too easy to say eat less fat and add more carbs or starches or eat healthier fats and fewer starches but what about the real truth. Why do all of those nutrition experts, doctors and scientist don't tell you the real truth? And that is to eat less protein. Where did the Chinese in the rural part of China get the protein? They eat just white rice. What about rural part of India or Nepal? Where is protein there? I am not saying these people are as healthy as they can be, they are not eating optimal diets by a long shot but where is their protein deficiency? If you get most of the calories from rice surely by the American standard, you will be long gone from protein deficiency. However, guess what, these people are still there, and they do not have any, not just protein but any individual amino acid deficiency. So someone lied to you, and that someone is your regular MD and industry and government and FDA and all of them. These poor people that don't eat animal protein live a very long life, and they are very healthy. Well as long as they do not move to big cities to work in factories or moved to the west and increased their protein or in other words animal products consumption. Then they start to have all of chronic diseases that we have. So it has nothing to do with fat or carb levels they ate from plant sources. Just about the levels of complete animal proteins they ate. And that is the truth, the elephant in the living room, that no one like to talk or even mention.

Our metabolism is very efficient in converting carbs to fats and another way around, but when it comes to the protein, it is a whole different story. Proteins are unique macronutrients that are different from two others. Why is protein so different? It is because it contains an atom called nitrogen. All proteins have nitrogen in them. What is a big deal then with this nitrogen? Well, the body needs to do something with that nitrogen so that it can use protein as energy. What that nitrogen does it pollute the entire process sort of speak. We want to burn clean and remain toxin free. Nitrogen is a dirty byproduct that the body needs to deal with. Our cells don't need to be overburden with toxic byproducts of energy production. It will burden them and create damage. If we have too much nitrogen in our body, we will suffer toxic effects of it. We might don't fell the immediate pain, but the damage will be there. For comparison initially, you don't feel cancer cells growing inside you either. Even the most used textbook for students and in other areas on human physiology Guyton and Hall Textbook of Medical Physiology, when describing the obligatory use of protein, even there they say from 25 to 35 gram of protein a day just to stay even. And that is when you eat three times a day and don't do a diet. If you are on a diet obligatory (just to stay even) amount of protein you need can come close to zero, and yes I am not kidding, I will give you a study to read later. But why you need obligatory 25 grams of protein according to the Guyton and Hall Textbook of Medical Physiology that you will find in every medical school.

Well, you maybe don't know this but now we will have a lesson in human physiology just like in the college. I already mention the mechanism known as autophagy (self-eating on ancient Greek). Imagine this, you don't lose any protein. Let me write this again, your body has evolutionarily adapted to save anything that it can be saved including your dead cells. Every cell that dies in your body no matter what it is, if it is not infectious, it will be recycled. You eat yourself every day. You even eat like a vampire you own blood. The color of the stool is a consequence of hemoglobin digestion. Any cells that die in your body will be recycled. A red blood cell, any other immune cell any organ cell and so on. Let me write this again for all of those let get some gains bodybuilders out there, you don't lose any protein, it just gets recycled over and over and over and over again until you die. Why book say obligatory 25 grams, well because you do lose some but only when you eat. If you do not eat, you don't lose anything but when you eat some of your own cells in the digestive tract will be lost. Your poop is the marker and when measured the average man of 150 pounds lose about 25 to 35 grams a day of his own protein from intestinal lining as a consequence of digestion of food or other factors. The average man will also lose some of the protein on the growth of nails, hair, and skin. But that is in a range of a couple of grams a day. That is accepted medical school line of thinking today.

Everything more than 25-gram needs to go to energy production, and there is your nitrogen. However, also I want to mention this, many indigenous people eat much less protein and live a full healthy life. So 25 grams that you will lose in excrement is for standard American unhealthy diet. Why are some indigenous people in Africa able to live their entire life on 15 to 20 grams of protein a day. The truth is, the healthier the diet, the less you lose. Recycling is the real answer. You eat less you recycle more. You eat more you lose more. Our body is smart, and it knows how to keep us in balance. When you read 25 to 35 grams, even that is extremely generous. In reality, we need even less than that. It would be best if you told this to your gym 200 grams of protein a day manipulated frat boys. Protein has a much more toxic effect on our body's that you can even believe. It can even give you cancer. However, wait proteus comes from ancient Greek and means the first or primary and everybody you know always told you that protein is one of the most important macronutrients. The scientist will tell you that every cell in your body is made of proteins and what is the result. The result is that we start to think that the more protein, the better and that we must consume it in a large amount and of course eat all the food products that have a high percentage of protein like meat and dairy.

However, if you recycle protein almost to the 100 percent extent and lose only a small amount then what is going to happen with all of that extra protein you eat. Your body does not need it, so it is going to be transformed into fat for later energy use. To make thing even worse proteins that are made of amino acids are one of the scarcest thing in nature, so our bodies have adapted special mechanisms to extremely well absorb all of the protein from food. More than 80 percent of protein in the food you eat is going to be absorbed, and that is because the amino acids are the one thing that our body actively absorbs. What does that mean? Well, it means our bodies will do anything that they can to absorb every amino acid they can. In contrast minerals, for example, are passively absorbed into the bloodstream. They are just going thru the intestines, and our body does nothing except letting some of them naturally pass through the inner line. They have a hard time being absorbed. It is because in nature in normal conditions millions of years ago food was filled with minerals, and our bodies didn't need to develop any mechanism for mineral absorption. They even compete with each other for absorption, and our body's do nothing to absorb them. Minerals through diffusion only are absorbed into the circulation. However, now when we eat produce from land that is mineral deficient and only has a small number of minerals that are from artificially dropped fertilizers and we do not have a mechanism for mineral absorption but have all of the animal products we can eat the situation is going to be bad. We will have an abundance of protein in our diet like never before and lack of most of the minerals we need. We are now completely deficient in most of the trace minerals and some of the essential minerals as well and at the same time overburden with too much pro-actively absorbed protein.

Scarcity is the rule of protein in nature. Now how much protein, for example, one cup of kale has? It has 5 grams of protein. And these protein is complete as any animal protein or any other complete protein you can imagine. There is no such an entity as an incomplete protein. Every protein on earth from any food source has all essential amino acids. When there is conversation about the completeness of protein, it is actually a conversation about similarities of the source of the protein to our own. Every protein has all essential amino acids but in different proportions. "Completeness" is a word in medicine that is used to describe how much of proportion of amino acids in the protein that we are consuming match the proportion of amino acids in our own cells. As long as you eat more than two different things in your life. The entire story about the completeness of protein is a complete lie. Every food you eat and that is correct will have a different profile of amino acids. If you eat different foods, you will get different profiles of amino acids and what is that called? It is called complete protein. Why? Because our body has a reserve, a pull of essential amino acids that is filled with various essential amino acids when they are in excess.

Some food products have high levels of all essential amino acids in them. That will be all proteins from the animal kingdom. So all proteins that are from eggs, meat and dairy are "complete." Meat is meat and protein is similar in proportions of amino acids that it has. Some of the plant sources have "complete" protein like soy for example. Eating complete protein is not a good idea because it will raise the levels of IGF-1 hormone and that is not something you want. IGF-1 is cancer promoting hormone. There is a greater link between IGF-1 level and overall cancer then between smoking and lung cancer for example. That is a hormone that basically goes around your body and let say it this way knock on the cell door. When lady of the house opens the door's IGF-1 will say: "Hello, how are you doing fine lady, I just come by to say to you that if you need to divide or repair something in your house we have all of the essential amino acids in the street right now ". The response from a normal cell will be: "No thank you we are ok, and everything is fine," but cancer cell will just say: "Thank you, sir, let's have a dividing party." Chronically elevated levels of IGF-1 is not something anybody as an adult person should want, including bodybuilders. Most of the studies find no correlation between protein intake and IGF-1 and that will be a response from your doctor and industry.

However, guess what, it is one more lie. These studies did not take into account animal versus plant protein. In this study (The Associations of Diet with Serum Insulin-like Growth Factor I and Its Main Binding Proteins in 292 Women Meat-Eaters, Vegetarians, and Vegans; Naomi E. Allen, Paul N. Appleby, Gwyneth

K. Davey, Rudolf Kaaks, Sabina Rinaldi and Timothy J. Key) they did exactly that. Higher IGF-1 levels were only associated with eating complete protein, meaning all of the animal protein but also soy protein as well. Actually, plant protein seems to decrease the levels of IGF-1. The conclusion was that it is not the excessive protein in general that raises the cancer-promoting IGF-1 level but only complete protein. IGF 1 is so bad that it is not only that it helps all types of cancer to grow but it also helps them to break off from the main tumor and migrate to bloodstream and other parts of the body creating metastatic tumor cells (Growth Hormone and Insulin-Like Growth Factor-I in the Transition from Normal Mammary Development to Preneoplastic Mammary Lesions doi.org/10.1210/er.2008-0022). It is not a tumor that will kill you in 95 percent of the cases it is metastatic tumors all over the body. What help breast cancer cell to migrate to the liver, bone, brain, lung. It is IGF-1 (Growth Factors and their receptors in cancer metastases. Front Biosci (Landmark Ed). 2011 Jan 1;16:531-8).

There is rare genetic mutation a syndrome that some people have that creates a form of dwarfism as a consequence of the low level of IGF-1 creation. It is called a Laron Syndrome. They never, let me write this again, they never get cancer (Growth hormone receptor deficiency is associated with a major reduction in pro-aging signaling, cancer, and diabetes in humans. doi: 10.1126/scitranslmed.3001845). In this study cancer death rate in these people was zero. Not just that they tent to live much longer. Vegans also tend to live longer them meat eaters and even when we look at animal kingdom. Plant-eating species ten to live longer than carnivores. In 1993 there was a great breakthrough in the science of longevity. To date, it was a study that managed to prolong the life of specific species of roundworm to double the amount. It was so far the longest recorded life extension in any study. There was one mutation that was found that had doubled the life expectancy of roundworms from 30 to 60 days (A C. elegans mutant that lives twice as long as wild-type. Nature. 1993 Dec 2;366(6454):461-4.). It was as same as people would live for 160 years and be healthy. And it was just one single mutation that did that much. When we consider a topic of aging, we think of telomere length, DNA free radical damage, multiple other processes and so on. But no it was just one single mutation that did only one thing. That one gene scientist named Grim Reaper gene and it was just malfunction in IGF-1 receptor gene. If you eat animal protein, you do not just expose yourself to cancer risk but also speed up the aging process. Science today can create artificial retroviruses that can cause mutations. In the future, it might be plausible to have a vaccine that will deactivate the IGF-1 receptor in adult humans to some extent and prolong our life for double the amount but for now just avoid animal protein.

When we switch people to eat plant-based, we can significantly lower the levels of IGF-1 in the bloodstream. In one study the result was that people eating for 14 years plant-based diet had half the levels of IGF-1 in the bloodstream then meat-eaters (Effect of diet and exercise on serum insulin, IGF-I, and IGFBP-1 levels and growth of LNCaP cells in vitro (United States). Cancer Causes Control. 2002 Dec;13(10):929-35). And you have to be a vegan not vegetarian. In this study they compared the IGF-1 levels of vegans, lacto ovo vegetarians and meat eaters and only vegans had lower circulation IGF-1 level (The Associations of Diet with Serum Insulin-like Growth Factor I and Its Main Binding Proteins in 292 Women Meat-Eaters, Vegetarians, and Vegans; Naomi E. Allen, Paul N. Appleby, Gwyneth K. Davey, Rudolf Kaaks, Sabina Rinaldi and Timothy J. Key DOI: Published November 2002). Milk and eggs are still complete animal proteins, so the result is understandable. This was a study on a woman, but later studies on men and woman showed the same thing. In one study they compared the statistic correlation between smoking and lung cancer and high animal protein consumption and overall cancer risk and the correlation was even worse for the protein (Low protein intake is associated with a major reduction in IGF-1, cancer, and overall mortality in the 65 and younger but not older population. doi: 10.1016/j.cmet.2014.02.006). This was a recent study done in 2014 with the conclusion:" Mice and humans with growth hormone receptor/IGF-1 deficiencies display major reductions in age-related diseases. Because protein restriction reduces GHR-IGF-1 activity, we examined links between protein intake and mortality. Respondents aged 50-65 reporting high protein intake had a 75% increase in overall mortality and a 4-fold increase in cancer death risk during the following 18 years." When you eat animal protein you have four times more chance to develop cancer. When you smoke, you have four-time also more chance to develop lung cancer. Then add toxic overload into the picture and if you are meat eater that also smoke and lives generally like most of the Americans then the situation is going to be as it is. One of three people are going to die from cancer. Some of the press wrote about this study creating widespread anger among medical practice and also among the general population as well. What was the response from the medical community? Gunter Kuhnle, a food nutrition scientist not some regular but specifically nutrition scientist at Reading University, said: "It was wrong and potentially even dangerous to compare the effects of smoking with the effect of meat and cheese as the study does. Sending out [press] statements such as this can damage the effectiveness of important public health messages. They can help to prevent sound health advice from getting through to the general public. The smoker thinks: Why to bother quitting smoking if my cheese and ham sandwich is just as bad for me."

The real message is that the cancer epidemic is caused by animal protein. Or let be precise here complete protein in general. The real message is don't eat animal protein there is enough protein in plants. Actually, all the protein ever created on planet earth is created by plants. All essential proteins are in the plants first, and animals get them after eating plants. Animals only grow by eating plants that have made all of the essential proteins. Then some predators eat other animals and so on. Remember that all essential amino acids, all protein on the entire planet were made by and only by plants. Only one actually incomplete protein in the entire food supply is gelatin. So only and only one protein source we could not live on is jello. On the other hand, there is only one truly perfect protein for us not counting mothers milk. The highest quality protein on the planet for us is our own human flesh. Although we do not practice cannibalism anymore there is evidence we ate Neanderthals and other primates, so we practice a form of fellow mammal's cannibalism. We do not like anything out of the mammalian kingdom to much like insects or reptiles. We prefer our own. It is all because we need that protein. Or how about this. Did you know that beans have as much protein as regular meat with zero cholesterol, saturated fat, dead bacteria endotoxins, and are full of fiber antioxidants and resistant starch? This entire concept that there is somehow incomplete protein and that plant protein is inferior to an animal is just another lie designed and produced by the same people that use science as a tool for marketing. The lie we accept and use as justification for our own desire for the animal flesh.

The real truth is that in entire medical practice history so far there was not one single case of protein deficiency recorded. There are millions of people dying from calorie deficiency meaning regular hunger but protein deficiency no. Does not exist. There is only one case in veterinary practice when they feed cows with corn that lack one specific amino acid. There is 0.02 g amount of Tryptophan (Trp) standard amino acid in 100 g, grams portion amount of Corn, and corn is not regular cow food so low levels of Tryptophan in cattle diet can make them restless because the brain is using Tryptophan to make serotonin, a happiness hormone. A corn diet is a diet that will make cattle depressed. That is the only case of amino acid deficiency that I know about. This entire story about lacking amino acids and completeness is just a marketing myth, and I am not kidding. It started on February 75 issue of Vogue magazine were some paid scientist made a recommendation that combining different plant proteins we can create a complete one that our bodies need. "Complementary proteins" myth was born and is still well alive and kicking. So what now, you still think plant proteins are not as good, you need to eat complete protein from animal sources or at least do complementary proteins combining. Our own body evolved not to be stupid. We have a reserve pool of all essential amino acids disregarding almost 90 grams of proteins that our bodies recycle every day. Even if you want to design a study with the diet from whole plant foods that will be sufficient in calories but insufficient in protein, it would be scientifically impossible. We can survive just eating rice or potatoes and nothing else indefinitely. There might be some other nutrition deficit but protein or any particular amino acid no. Even carrot juice has 2 percent of protein making it a sufficient for survival.

What you need to do is forget about protein. Forget that it exists. It is just a marketing scam. You will never be deficient in protein even if you are on fruitarian diet. We and almost half of the planet to recently ate nothing but the rice and had never been protein deficient. Still, you think the protein is important. Ok, what will happen if you don't eat it for an entire year at all? You have obligatory 25 grams you need, that is what conventional medical science is telling us now. What would happen if you do not eat any amount of protein for an entire year, not one gram of it? By the way, 100 grams of tissue is not 100 grams of protein, it is about 22 to 25. Rest of it is water and fat. So if you do not eat protein for a year and do water fasting would you lose normal tissue beside fat as conventional medical science seems to propose. The answer is no. You will only lose fat and only initially some small amount of tissue.

And now I know I am going against entire Western Civilization so let us remember one study I already mention in part 1 of the series. Do you remember the morbidly obese 27-year-old Scottish man who water fasted for an entire year under medical supervision (Features of a successful therapeutic fast of 382 days duration, Postgrad Med J. 1973 Mar; 49(569): 203–209). He was given vitamin supplements daily. From day 93 to day 162, he was given potassium and from day 345 to day 355 only he was given 2.5 g of table salt daily. No other drug treatment was given. However, wait where is the protein? Where are obligatory 25 grams of it? The patient lost 276 pounds during his 382 days of dieting but wait how is he still alive? According to medical science obligatory protein is the must. How many pounds of muscle tissue did he lose if 25 grams of obligatory protein is 100 grams of normal tissue? Well, he did not lose any of the muscle or tissue at all. He just lost fat, and the protein got recycled for an entire year. He might have lost some of the muscle, but that is it. So let me ask again. How much protein do we need to eat to live? How about the quality or completeness of the protein?

The entire myth of protein quality was made from one rodent study done more than a hundred years ago that found that infant rats do not grow as well on plant as much as animal protein. Yes, I am not kidding that was one the study that have grown into a myth about protein completeness. Infant rats, by the way, don't grow well on human milk either because human milk has ten time less protein then rats milk. Rat milk has so much protein in it because the rats grow fast and human babies do not. The more protein in milk the faster the species is growing. How much protein do you think human breast milk has? Human milk has 9.5 gram of protein per one liter. Rat milk has 86.9 grams of protein per liter. Human breast milk has the lowest protein percentage from all in existence mammalian milks. Less than 1 percent protein by weight. What bodybuilders really should do is to find and drink some rats milk. That will grow the muscle no need for a whey protein supplement. What about vegan bodybuilding, or what about vegetarians or what about everyone? How much protein, in reality, do the different types of diets have? In this study (Nutrient profiles of vegetarian and nonvegetarian dietary patterns, doi: 10.1016/j.jand.2013.06.349.) they analyzed the average intake of protein comparing different diets. It was the largest study of this kind to date. They compared nutrient diet profiles of about 5,000 vegans, 30,000 standards all you desire meat eaters, flexitarians, 20,000 vegetarians, then divided them into groups from lacto-ovo, pesco to strict and semi and so on. The result is that all of the groups average about the same, around 60 for strict vegans to 90 grams for standard meat eater of proteins a day. Except that nonvegetarians had the lowest intakes of phytochemicals and antioxidant and fiber, beta-carotene, and magnesium with the highest intakes of cholesterol, toxins of all kind and saturated, trans, arachidonic, and docosahexaenoic fatty acids. If we ask the natural science of today, the consensus is that at the most you need 0.8 to 0.9 of grams of protein per kilogram and not counting all of the excess fat in obese people. Just fat-free body weight (Identifying recommended dietary allowances for protein and amino acids: a critique of 2007 WHO/FAO/UNU report. doi: 10.1017/S0007114512002450).

It is more likely that we will suffer from excess of protein that can cause a wide range of problems from increased cancer risk, precipitated progression of coronary artery disease, disorders of liver function, disorders of renal function, disorders of bone and calcium homeostasis (Adverse Effects Associated with Protein Intake above the Recommended Dietary Allowance for Adults. doi: 10.5402/2013/126929). The best thing to do is I will write this again, forget that you have ever heard the word protein. Start thinking mineral deficiencies, start thinking fiber start thinking antioxidant deficiencies. Green leafy vegetables are not considered a good source of protein by whom? The cattle industry. What about minerals? Do green leafy vegetables have abundant levels of minerals in them so that we do not need to develop special mechanisms to try to absorb them actively? We have shifted our diet, and that is exactly what we can see in the average population. An overabundance of cancer-promoting and toxifying proteins and deficiency in minerals and fiber in around 97 percent of the American population. Too much protein, too little minerals, and phytochemicals and fiber because in the past our diet was 97 percent plant-based 3 percent animal based.

High protein diet just burns protein into energy for storage. The end result is acid formation. Lactic acid, acidic acid, beta-Hydroxybutyric acid, sulfuric acid, phosphoric acid. These are all the acids that occur after excess protein degradation for energy storage. Burning or metabolizing excess protein is acid forming. Chronic kidney disease is a major problem affecting around 13 percent of the US population. When we compare the diet that was eaten by hominins the contemporary standard American diet is rich in saturated fat, simple sugars, filled with cholesterol and so on and in an essence is just the acid producing diet. Our ancestors evolved on the alkaline-producing diet. Our ancestors eat plant based alkaline diet, and we are eating animal product protein rich acid diet. So where did all of that acid goes at the end? It goes to the kidneys for neutralization by minerals especially calcium. Animal protein acid diet is believed to impact kidney function by tubular toxicity of elevated ammonium of the renin-angiotensin system. Ammonia is a base, so kidneys create ammonia to neutralize all the acid from excess protein. In the long turn, ammonia intratubular concentration rises to cause inflammation and kidney damage. Also acid creates a production of free radicals and damage everything in the entire body including kidneys. Excess protein coming from a whole food plant source should at least have some antioxidants in the food package to fight some of that inflammation.

Animal protein is just bad, no antioxidants but dead bacteria load of inflammatory endotoxins and saturated fat and cholesterol. Also at least to some extent plant protein is less acid forming as it tends to have less of sulfur-containing amino acids than animal one. Acid is generated by metabolism of organic sulfur in dietary protein. If you have chronic kidney disease, you need to go vegan and lower the overall protein intake to a 25 to 30 gram per day amount. It is standard medical therapy for decades with patients that have chronic kidney failure. If we look at people above 65 years of age one in three has chronic kidney disease. After the year 40, there is a slow decline in kidney function due to all ammonia damage so by the year of 65, 1 in 3 are seriously ill. The majority of these kidney disease patients do not progress to go to dialysis because they die first. Older adults with kidney disease have a fear of dialysis, but they are 13 times more likely to go underground before that happens from other diseases like heart attacks and strokes and so on. A plant-based diet is the only option for this kind of patients because plant based low protein diet help with protection against kidney inflammation, cancer and stones, acidosis as well, and also is beneficial for the cardiovascular system by reducing cholesterol and chronic inflammation and so on. The only thing worse for the kidneys then animal protein is saturated fat and cholesterol. They can directly kill kidney cells by clogging them and poking holes in them. In regular medicine, it has been acknowledged for a very long period that cholesterol and animal or to be precise saturated fat have a direct toxic effect on kidneys (Lipid nephrotoxicity in chronic progressive glomerular and tubulointerstitial disease; Lancet. 1982 Dec 11;2(8311):1309-11). Low protein vegan diet is the only treatment for such patients (Potential benefits of renal diets on cardiovascular risk factors in chronic kidney disease patients. Ren Fail. 2007;29(5):529-34.).

Again the problem is an abrupt shift in our diet and lifestyle. We all have genes telling our body to absorb as much protein as it can because it was so scarce in nature and today despite the extreme surplus we are going to absorb every amino acid we can. It had become one more maladaptation to our current standard American diet. And we get poisoned by it, and that is secret they do not want to tell you. Even people who are health oriented or even vegans are still brainwashed to think they need to get that protein, or they are going to die or get some disease. Well just tell that to the Scottish man that didn't eat one gram of it for the entire year. There is one more myth we need to debunk. For a long period of time to almost a couple of year ago, there was a myth that excess protein acidosis is neutralized by calcium. That is correct so where does the body take the calcium from? Well, the bones of course. There was a belief that lasted for a long time that over excessive protein intake is going to leach out calcium from the bones. If you eat high protein meal calcium level in urine rises. Add meat to the diet, and we have a significant calcium loss through urine. If meat and eggs have five times more sulfur containing amino acids, then plant based protein that will create acidosis. The body will buffer it by calcium, and we will have calcium loss. People with osteoporosis are told to avoid high protein diet. For every 40 grams of protein, we are going to pee out about 50 mg of calcium which is 2 percent of complete bone mass loss in one year and leading to osteoporosis. It was not until this study (The impact of dietary protein on calcium absorption and kinetic measures of bone turnover in women. J Clin Endocrinol Metab. 2005 Jan;90(1):26-31.) that calcium loss is found to be coming from increased absorption from food. Protein seems to boost calcium absorption. They gave radioactive calcium in food and measured to see if calcium loss in urine is radioactive. It turned out to be radioactive too. That means extra calcium is coming from food and high-protein diets are not detrimental to bone. Other studies have been done from that time and supported this new finding.

However, it is not just calcium that is used to buffer all the acids. Other minerals are used to, and it seems by some number of studies done so far that muscle tissue is the source of minerals, not bone calcium. Alkaline diet might be protective against muscle loss (Alkaline diets favor lean tissue mass in older adults doi: [10.1093/ajcn/87.3.662]). In any case, high protein especially high protein from an animal source is not our natural and healthy diet no matter what paleo people say. However, brainwashing is brainwashing. In this study that I already mention (Nutrient profiles of vegetarian and nonvegetarian dietary patterns, doi: 10.1016/j.jand.2013.06.349) you will see that vegan's, vegetarians and all other groups tested in the study all have almost the same amount of excess protein intake. It is because of the regular medical, and Big Pharma industry has an active interest to manipulate you so that they can sell you all of their products and drugs. So why don't you go and eat that protein you so desire, and of course that whey powder and the more, the better? And of course, you need to be apologetic and excuse yourself if you do not eat that much protein and tell people you are getting your protein from more beans and nuts and soy. You need to be self-conscious and feel bad and have neurotic tendencies when protein is mentioned because you are brainwashed by design. Even doctors are thought to force the brainwashing and ask vegans and even vegetarians about their protein intake. In real reality, 99 percent of Americans eat flesh and are chronically diseased to the maximum level, but you need to get that protein, or else. Now there are even bags of vegan protein that they sell, not just whey anymore. High protein bar and snacks. Every time I hear people in the gym or anywhere else talking about protein I know that they don't know anything about nutrition even nutritionist and regular MDs.

Just forget about protein. Remember that 25 was obligatory for what we lose in a stool and average vegan eats around 60. Forget that you ever heard the word protein. There is also a question if we used to get around 15 grams of protein in a day and many indigenous populations until recently still did get to that number on average how is it that vegans today get 60. It is because of a higher quality of the diet. We would never be able to get to eat an entire ball of beans or nuts or seeds in the amount we can do today. We had been eating more starch-based USO and regular vegetables then average vegan eats today. Today average vegan eats much more of high protein plant-based products like beans, nuts, seeds and so on then it was common in the evolution of the species. As a result, we get much more protein then we did. Even as a strict vegan. Now our bodies today can deal from protein toxicity to some degree. Animal protein is much worse, but for vegans, it is still some of the concern, but somehow our bodies can handle 60 grams of plant-based protein a day without too much of a damage. Most of the damage comes from nitrogen. When you cut out nitrogen from amino acids, it creates new substances. For instance, ammonia is one of them, and it is very toxic.

There is a creation of nitrogen-based free radicals that our body does not handle very well or does not handle as well as oxygen free radicals. Burning of sugar and fat creates oxygen-based free radicals that we can handle, but now we have all that excess of protein and nitrogen-based free radicals as a result that our bodies cannot handle. And these nitrogen free radicals stick with us and do damage everywhere, and every time we eat fatty foods those nitrogen-based free radicals are going to react with them in the body turning them into rancid fats. Bodybuilder eats at average more than 200 grams of protein per day. Physiologically it is not possible to grow more than 10 grams of protein per day (which is around 50 grams of tissue) if you are not on steroids no matter how much protein you eat or how much you exercise. Even strict vegan can do bodybuilding if a protein is an issue. Other types of athletes usually eat much more than average amounts also. Some keto paleo health advocates will eat 10 eggs for breakfast. To some people, they are health gurus.

There is a trend to eat large amounts of complete protein to lose weight. The logic behind it is that a large amount of complete protein will stimulate the larger release of IGF-1 hormone that will stop the autophagy of the muscle mass and only focus the weight loss on fat tissue. And that argument is correct. It is scientifically proven, and you can eat a large amount of complete protein on dieting to stop autophagy of muscle tissue by some extent. However, do you want cancer as a result of looking good? The real question here is not where do you get your protein but how to avoid the excess. Especially how to avoid an excess of animal protein. Why animal protein is not good for species that are not carnivorous by nature and have low acidity is because even if you cook protein low acidity in our stomachs might don't break up animal protein completely. Protein is made out of the chain of amino acids. That what protein is. Different amino acids bind together in chains to form globular protein. Some proteins can have hundreds of amino acids bound together that not even the enzymes can go through them. These large globular proteins are hard to digest for us because again we have low acidity. Green leafy vegetables have the simplest forms of proteins almost couple of amino acids just bound together. Beans and especially nuts and seeds can have vast complex harder to digest proteins. Animal protein is the most complex with the most amino acids in the chain. What happens when you don't break up completely these globular proteins. Some of them end up in bloodstream eventually, especially if you have leaky gut or some inflammation in intestines. As soon as there are amino acids that are not in single form but bound together that means we have an organism that is invading us. That is what our immune system thinks when it detects amino acids in chains going thru the bloodstream. Then what happens is that the immune system makes an antibody to that globular chain of amino acids to kill that invader. Now if you have leaky gut and you eat a lot of plant protein and some of them end up in the bloodstream, and you have an immune reaction it will just give you inflammation or allergy.

However, what happens when you eat animal protein? What happens is that animal protein can be similar to our own. In a sense all animals have similar organs. If by any chance a sequence of amino acids is the same as the sequence of amino acids in some of our own cells after the antibody is created to deal with that invader it will detect the same amino acid sequence in our own cells and our own immune system will start to attack our own cells thinking they are still some invading microorganism. That is how every autoimmune disease starts. As an infection or inflammation because of molecular mimicry. All because we have leaky gut and low acid to properly digest globular animal proteins that we should not be eating in the first place. If immune system had made the antibody that will attack our own cells there is no cure anymore. Autoimmune diseases are not genetic; they are just one more example of maladaptation. If the right conditions are met, anybody can get them. Autoimmune diseases are the worst nightmare you can imagine. If you consume too many nuts and seeds, you might have some digestive dysfunction, but that is it. Globular hard to digest plant proteins can only give you allergies. When you see the writing on a food product where it says does not contain soy, dairy, eggs, gluten, peanut and so on. It is because these are all hard to digest globular proteins that some people have immune reactions to. We should not overeat hard to digest globular protein on day to day basis because it can cause inflammation and then food allergies and in worst case scenario some form of autoimmune disease. In nature, in natural evolution, we would be exposed to flaxseed for example once a year. We would not be eating them on a regular everyday basis. That is why I suggest to people to have a variety in the diet and to avoid eating excessive amounts of hard to digest globular proteins especially if they are from the animal source. Everyone in my view should do a food sensitivity testing to know what food to avoid. Some might have a problem with gluten some with peanuts some can eat anything and do not have an immune reaction, but you need to test it. You might have a food sensitivity, not allergy, and you might don't even know it.

Now let us talk about a big secret. The one they do not want you to know about. The one that is so important that they do not want even to mention the name of it. The big secret of what causes an epidemic of cancer. One of the biggest industries in the world. Or let say it this way. You have not been told the truth about cancer. Cancer is not even the disease at all. You cannot get infected by it. Maybe with bio-weaponized sv40 you might, but not in normal conditions. It is more state or condition of the body that is malfunctioning. Medical science had known for decades what is underlying this condition but have done everything in their power not to tell the whole truth. If I know and I am not a scientist, then I am pretty sure that real scientists know, just are doing everything they can to find a drug or cure for cancer that they can charge. But not even that is the truth. They will never really heal you. They will treat you and you will have to come back to pay for some more treatments later until all of your life savings are gone, and then you can go too. They do not care. What they teach to the future oncologist or when you pick up a regular collage oncology book in any of the bookstores and look on what is cancer definition this is what they will like you to believe. For example, this is what is written in the American Cancer Society cancer book: "Although most of us think cancer is a single disease it is actually a family of more than a hundred different types." Ok, what is this even mean. What is this that they and when I say they I mean the medical industry is telling you about cancer? They will first like you to be scared and confused because there are more than a million different types that can kill you and secondly they call cancer a disease that is not the real truth. Some virus that can attack you by infection is a real disease. Cancer is not an infection, so it is not a disease it is a condition. A huge difference here. It is a specific malfunctioning of the body, not a disease that you can pick up in public transportation. They call cancer: "a whole family of diseases." This is what we have been told for the last 70 years. This is what they teach in medical college. However, what real science is going to tell you is that basically, it is not more than 100 types of disease but just one type of condition. What real science is going to tell you is that cancer all of them are regular cells that have suffered a form of mutation of cellular genes. Cancer is caused in all instances by mutation. That is it.

Maybe you do not know this by right now you have cancer. I have cancer too. Every individual species on this planet has some percentage of cells that are mutated in some form. We all have cancer cells just our immune system deals with them. In normal condition, there will be one newly formed mutant cell on every few millions of regular cells. Body is built up of 75 trillion cells, so we have in normal condition a pretty large colony of cancer cells all the time. And when I say normal, I mean healthy vegan whole food diet and exercise living in a clean environment individual. The question here is if we all have large colonies of cancer cells and cancer is disease why all of us have not died from cancer? It is immune system and autophagy that eats up these cells before they overpopulate. That is the real truth. There is no: "a whole family of diseases" cancer industry half-truth myth. If immune system is down and is vastly outnumbered there is going to be a condition that will allow for a formation of cancer and the body can develop several different types of cancer depending on the individual condition. It is because whatever condition allows one cancer to overpopulate will allow some other types of cancer to form also again depending on individual condition. Only if the body is healthy and has very efficient immune system cancer cannot exist. What we need to do is to stop attacking cancer and start improving our own immune system and condition. The immune system will do it regular job by keeping cancer cells in normal number not allowing them to overpopulate and form a lump of tissue. Because when cancer forms a lump, it becomes whole another beast that tricks immune system not to recognize it by different methods. However, in normal condition individual or small cluster of cancer cells in our bodies are completely normal. Cancer is completely normal "disease" for the human condition in normal circumstances. We all have it as a part of our bodies normal functioning for our entire life. Cancer cells are not foreign object to our body, a foreign invader, so the entire Nixon let us declare war on cancer is illegal, but it did give a lot of money that were used to start the cancer industry. The industry that does nothing except prolonging the misery.

Until we understand that there is a big difference between a single condition and 100 different types of diseases we will not realize the truth. The real truth is that cancer is a single condition that can manifest itself in 100 different ways. Now that is the truth that they do not want to teach on medical college or tell the public. We are made up from 75 trillion cells, and we have more than 200 different cells in our body. So if we found a mutating cell in our colon it would be called colon cancer, if we found a mutating cell in our brain it would be called brain cancer, if we found a mutating cell in our bone it would be called bone cancer and so on. They way medical industry identify the "diseases" is misleading, or in other words, cancer is not named on what it is. It is named by the way that it is perceived to be by the individual that is looking at it from the outside. It is named on tissue from which they are made or where the cell was found or how fast they are growing. It can also be named by some famous athlete or person that had them or even by the name of the researcher that found it first and decided to name it after him. So you see we could have over 200 different "diseases" of cancer because we have over 200 different types of cells. One cancer for every cell.

The whey medical industry defend this argument is that by some extent the cancer cells take much of the characteristics of the cell that was mutated from not just the characteristics by the mutation itself. In a way, this is correct because there are completely different acting cancer cells depending on the source of mutation. Some are less dangerous or not dangerous at all. Some are almost 100 percent death sentence. However, this still does not make it the family of diseases. It is still just one same condition that manifested itself differently. Genetic predisposition can play a role, different environmental factors and so on. However, it is still in the base one singular condition. A misconstructed confused cell that does nothing except multiply or in the meantime waiting to be eaten up or destroyed. We hear the word attack all the time, cancer have attacked the liver, cancer have attacked this and that. Cancer is not bacteria that eat your tissue as food. It does not attack anything. It is just a confused cell that does what every cell does. Multiply. The problem is that in time it can multiply to be so large that it kills you. However, it is not in a medical sense attacking us as some virus does. The problem is the immune system that does nothing to prevent this because in some cases it does not recognize the mutated cell as a foreign invader. Cancer is not a disease in the purest form. It is a symptom of the inefficient immune system. You can think of it like something that is similar to the AIDS virus. That is the real truth about cancer.

Can we go and ask the medical profession to reclassify cancer? As long as we believe that cancer is disease, we will treat it like any other disease, and we will be in good service of modern medicine paying chemotherapy. Only when the immune system is incapable of destroying these malignant cells, and only then cancer will progress to be a full-blown "disease." For example, AIDS patients usually develop three types of extremely rare cancers; Non-Hodgkin lymphoma (NHL, also known as AIDS-related lymphoma or ARL), Kaposi's sarcoma, and cervical cancer. Forty percent of HIV+ patients develop one of those cancers. For people that do not know the immune system is much similar to the brain. It has the capacity for learning and storing memory and creating and storing and using information. Vaccines are dead viruses given to your immune system to "learn" how to deal with them later in life if the true active virus came. The immune system is learning all the time and is active all the time. Immune system malfunction when it stops attacking cancer cells is the real cause of the problem.

The treatment of cancer by strengthening the immune system is today almost universally suppressed. They do not want to prevent cancer and lower the rate to natural 2 percent of genetic causes and then try to heal that. No, they want to suppress the knowledge and represent the cancer as a disease that they need to treat with some magic cancer-killing drug that you are going to pay. How much did your life cost by the way? If you have cancer how much are you willing to spend on treatments? What if your child has it? In some rare occasions, some of the regular researchers do get credited for telling the truth. For example, in 1989 two researchers from University of California San Francisco won Nobel Prize in medicine by discovering that cancer is not family of different diseases with causes that we do not understand, but Michael Bishop and Harold E. Varmus won it for their discovery of the cellular origin of retroviral oncogenes. In other words, they found that cancer is a single condition caused by oncogenes, a single unifying explanation of how cancer occurs. They published their research back in 1976, so for a long time the industry has known and did nothing to utilize this discovery in "war on cancer." Immunologists are not welcomed in any speech or research about cancer. Just oncologist that have learned what industry likes them to learn and they do chemo and radiation and other "nice" stuff to people for the last century.

There are a few studies done independently. There are some places that do that kind of research. Recent years it started to be little more accepted. Today there are even studies that did nutrition experiments on cancer research. However, it was done usually by rogue doctors like Dr. Dean Ornis or such a type of physicians that do not go with the line of the conventional cancer industry. I will reference some of the studies in this chapter.

So what will weaken the immune system? How about chronic inflammation as a consequence of inadequate diet that is filled with dead meat bacteria endotoxins and pesticides and hormones and toxic acidic protein byproducts that cause inflammation. How about lacking anti-inflammatory nutrients like antioxidants and other phytochemicals. How about toxic overload from environmental mutagens. How about lacking an adequate level of autophagy by constant overeating. To seal the deal, there is chronically elevated IGF-1 level from animal or let be a precise, complete protein. All the things that I have mentioned is a consequence of excessive animal protein in the diet. All of them except environmental mutagens. So what causes an epidemic of cancer? It is again maladaptation to our current diet and technologically shaped lifestyle. Are you going to get bone or brain cancer depends on individual genetic predisposition and many other environmental factors but then there is also reality that today in modern human civilization 1 in 3 individuals will die from cancer. That is an epidemic of biblical proportions caused by an abrupt shift in our lifestyle. The medical industry will dispute this but then go to nature. Ask yourself, are there any other species of primates that have such a high rate of cancer, or any other species in general? Monkeys can die from cancer but not in numbers of 1 in 3. It is not genetic. Genetic plays the role, but the underlying cause is maladaptation to current high-quality animal protein diet. About 2 percent of cancers are today by standard research and medicine considered to be purely caused by genetic factors. Only 2 percent is number given by conventional medicine. Rest of it is diet. Or to be more precise animal protein and toxic overload.

You still don't want to believe that animal protein is the initial cause of cancer. In this study (Effects of a low-fat, high-fiber diet and exercise program on breast cancer risk factors in vivo and tumor cell growth and apoptosis in vitro. Nutr Cancer. 2006;55(1):28-34.) they put woman on a low-fat (10-15% kcal), high-fiber (30-40 g per 1,000 kcal/day) diet meaning vegan and also forced them to do daily exercise classes for just 14 days. Serum insulin and IGF-1 were significantly reduced in all women. The conclusion was: " In vitro growth of the BCa cell lines was reduced by 6.6% for the MCF-7 cells, 9.9% for the ZR-75-1 cells, and 18.5% for the T-47D cells. Apoptosis was increased by 20% in the ZR-75-1 cells, 23% in the MCF-7 cells, and 30% in the T-47D cells (n = 12)." In translation just look at the image. They took some blood from a woman and dropped them on cancer cells. When you see all that white dots that is the cancer cell that is dead as a result. If you eat a regular diet, there was still some anti-cancer activity, and you can see that one spot on the petri dish to the left. This is what vegan blood does after 14 days.

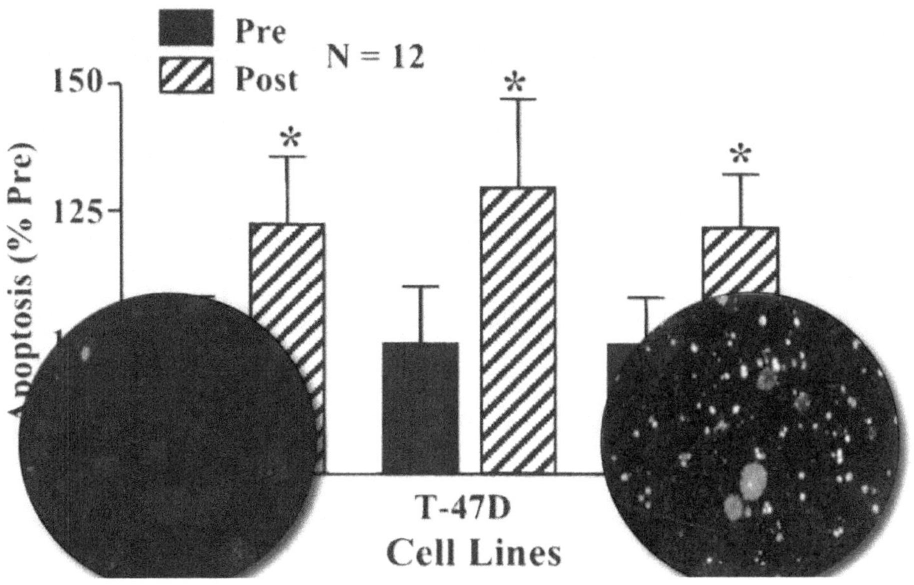

There was a similar experiment with men and prostate cancer with the result showing blood that kill cancer cells eight times better, and so far tens of different experiments with vegan diet and cancer and the result are always the same. Cause of cancer is standard American diet as a trigger to IGF-1 chronic elevation and all of the immune system inactivity due to all of the pollutant and toxic overload coming from the environment and diet. There were studies on a vegan diet, but then they added injectable IGF-1 to their bodies the same one the bodybuilders like to use, and the end result was that the blood killing potential of cancer cells in vitro was back to normal. Effect of lowering IGF-1 level to cancer growth was so remarkably powerful that in this study done by Dr. Dean Ornish (Intensive lifestyle changes may affect the progression of prostate cancer. J Urol. 2005 Sep;174(3):1065-9; discussion 1069-70.) they were able to slow down the progression of prostate cancer by a remarkable 8 times rate and I quote: "The growth of LNCaP prostate cancer cells (American Type Culture Collection, Manassas, Virginia) was inhibited almost 8 times more by serum from the experimental than from the control group (70% vs. 9%, p <0.001) ".

Food products and you need to remember this are a package deal. Proteins come with baggage. Animal protein with inflammation and cholesterol and fat and plant protein comes with antioxidant and fiber and does not raise the level of IGF-1. Some plants fight cancer so good that they are better than leading drugs with no side effects. You do not have to learn all of this just remember that variety is a key and if you want or have a family history of some form of cancer you can look up to some specific plants, mushrooms or supplements. Medicinal herbs and supplements are a vast topic, and I will analyze some of them like curcumin for instance in upcoming chapters in the book series.

Milk

"Milk is for babies. When you grow up you have to drink beer"

- Arnold Schwarzenegger

The media and the world tell us that milk is essential, and that cannot be a substituted, it is one of the vital food items, but let's look at some interesting facts.

If you have one ordinary wild cow, as it is one that lives in the plains in Africa, then such a cow will produce 3 liters of milk per day. That is enough to nourish its calf, and of course, this calf is equipped to consume that milk. For calf, there is no more natural food than that. The protein in milk is named Casein. It is large globular protein not like the one found in vegetables. It needs a particular digestion mode to be absorbed correctly. He needs a particular enzyme called renin so that the body can dissolve it to amino acids. Without this enzyme renin, it cannot be utilized. It will go just past the digestive system unabsorbed as a globular protein. The body absorbs only individual amino acids after the protein is broken down in the digestive tract. The calf will produce this enzyme in adequate amounts.

When we approach the business model of today economics that translate into "let's make more money", we will select cows for milking that are genetically conditioned to produce more milk in a day. Much more milk than wild cows. So good cow will produce 20 liters of milk per day, and a very good cow will produce 40 liters of milk per day, an excellent cow will produce 80 liters. The World Champion has produced over 120 liters a day.

We have to have a milk in our diet, as story goes, because of the facts that milk is primarily rich in calcium and proteins. Then about fat and lactose and other bad things in it, media do not speak much. They say that we consume our daily dose of calcium and protein primarily from milk. It is all about that calcium we need and proteins. We have been taught since the day we were babies to take the necessary doses of dairy products, milk, yogurts cheese so that we can grow. However, what science tells us is that our own human milk has the lowest concentration of proteins and the lowest proportion of the casein to whey from all mammals. Why does human milk have the lowest concentration of proteins from all mammals? The casein to each species is uniquely suited to meet the metabolic needs of that species, which means that it will have a specific amino acid composition, and the amount of protein in milk will be adjusted to the growing needs of that organism. It's 10g / l in human milk, and it takes 120 days for an infant to double its weight with growth, now horses have 24g / l, which is twice as much and it takes 60 days to double their weight, the cow is 33g / l and It takes only 47 days for calf to double its weight, the dog is 71g / l and only 8 days, rats 86.9 g /l and only 4.5 days and so on. If the casein is what we want the best source would be to milk rats.

Now let's think a little about this for a moment. If you are a rat, you need to grow rapidly to survive. If you are a rat, you need all that protein, and that is normal. However, why would the grow up human need all of that protein from the milk? So that we can get cancer and shorten our life from excessive IGF-1 and have diabetes and heart attack from all of that saturated fat. When there is a doubling of the weight of the calf in 47 days that is because of evolutionary reasons for its survival. The calf needs to strengthen fast, and it only takes a few hours on the same day when its born to start walking. It has to do so because many predators are lurking around and calf needs to be big and strong as soon as possible to survive. It grows rapidly because it has many natural predators, so energy in calves goes into the development of muscles, and for the development of muscles, it has a high dose of protein in milk during growth. A human baby is working hard and take much time to make the first step. A human baby needs constant care and is helpless and is growing so slowly in relation to the calf. What is the crucial thing for a human baby, a rapid growth of muscles? How about the brain. When the baby is born a head still has not closed fountains, and then the brain must develop very rapidly. Even the nerve endings are not entirely formed after birth, so brain needs food to develop. One day a cow will not be interested in mathematics, but a human might. What kind of food is necessary for the brain to develop? Answer is the fats. Most of your brain tissue consists of fat. There is a much higher fat ratio in human milk in relation to a protein that is perfect for brain development. The cow has a perfect relationship for the development of muscles. Now you can understand why children who are raised on cow's milk instead of their mother milk might have lower intelligence coefficients. There are studies done on this and not just one but hundreds of them. It is a well-documented fact in medicine that children fed with any other milk then mothers milk have lower IQ at an average level.

Also feeding infants with cow's milk leads to 80% probability of getting diarrhea, 70% probability of an outbreak of ear infections compared to infants nourished with mother's milk (A longitudinal analysis of infant morbidity and the extent of breastfeeding in the United States. Pediatrics. 1997 Jun;99(6):E5.). Babies fed with cow's milk during the other six months of life have a 30% increase in blood loss in internal organs and a significant loss of iron in their stool and low intakes of iron in general, linoleic acid, and vitamin E, and excessive intakes of sodium, potassium, and protein (Journal of Pediatrics, 1992; 89 (6): 1105-1109). So why is that? The problem is casein. You see cows have renin, but babies have very little to none of the renin, so they do not tolerate that protein. In breast milk there is naturally found bacterium Bacillus bifidus, which helps to dissolve casein from human milk. Cow milk in the child causes acidity, and also in adults, and irritates the intestines so that the intestines start to bleed. In addition to this, even the magazine of the scientific dairy industry will say that milk raises the level of cholesterol. Milk fat is identified as fat because it contains cholesterol and is primarily saturated (Journal of Dairy Science, 1991; 74 (11): 4002-4012). Milk is good for rising cholesterol level. For lack of iron that occurs due to bleeding in the digestive organs and diabetes (Cow milk and insulin-dependent diabetes mellitus: is there a relationship? Am J Clin Nutr. 1990 Mar;51(3):489-91). There are well-known studies from Harvard, about ovarian cancer and of course, I will quote the famous British Magazine Lancet (Galactose consumption and metabolism in relation to the risk of ovarian cancer Lancet. 1989 Jul 8;2(8654):66-71). Then cataracts, (Digestive Diseases and Sciences, 1982: 257-64), and intolerance to lactose, and food allergies, and toxins. The is one thing that milk is supposedly good for, the osteoporosis. In reality milk actually worsens the symptoms of disease. Diabetes type 1 have long known to be caused by cow's milk. Today we know that even in mothers that drink cow's milk while their children are still breastfeeding can also produce this disease in their children. Research have discovered that if a mother drinks milk, then partially digested casein can end up in the bloodstream and then end up in mother's milk too. Our bodies cannot get rid of that globular protein if it enters the bloodstream, so it gets thrown out everywhere including mothers milk.

The famous medical journal Lancet published in 1999 that new evidence favors a controversial theory that feeding cow's milk to the babies causes the development of diabetes type 1 in later life. Why cow milk and how can it cause diabetes? Medical practice and regular science first said that cow's milk could not in any way be the cause of diabetes because Japanese who are like any other Asian population lactose intolerant also breastfeed babies but also develop type 1 diabetes. Not type 2, type 2 is a lifestyle disease, type 1 is an autoimmune disease. Then they discovered that Japanese babies that do get it belonged to mothers who adopted western eating habits, so they examined their mother's milk, and what they found was cow's casein. Now cow's casein is specific to cows, but there is an amino acid sequence in one part of the casein (A1 beta-casein) that turned out to be the same as the amino acid sequence in beta cells in the pancreas. The immune system will remove this toxic A1 beta-casein. It has on the brain a form of opioid effect and which is associated with the entire spectrum of the diseases and occurs due to mutation in cows. Otherwise all other mammals that exist including people and some regular non-mutant cows that are being milked in Australia and the New Zeeland have the form of standard A2 type of beta-casein.

What happens is that we cannot digest the casein properly. We cannot do what is natural for the calf because they have adequate levels of this enzyme in theirs body. There's no renin in cow's milk. Because human milk has so little protein human baby does not need to have all that renin. All adults have difficulty in the digestion of the casein also. So if you put the plant protein into your stomach, the digestion will end in 4 hours; if you eat meat digestion will end in 6 hours. Put the casein in your stomach, it will swell for 12 hours!! The Germans have a saying that the cheese closes the stomach, why? Because the stomach has trouble digesting casein. What happens is that from time to time stomach will open gaps to let some of the milk protein to intestine when the body accumulates some more of this enzyme. Then the stomach is closed again. Bodybuilders like to drink casein powder protein before bedtime because of this effect so that they have protein in the bloodstream all night long. Slow digestion is a consequence of lacking evolutionary adaptation to milk drinking. If you have a leaky gut or some intestine inflammation this protein will partially be immersed in the bloodstream. And now suddenly you have foreign proteins in your body. And what is a response from the immune system? The immune system is going to create the antibodies to fight this protein. And what happens when this protein has an unwanted amino acid chain. Now you have created an antibody that attacks this amino acid chain. If this chain is the same as in your beta cells, the antibody will attack them also. It will attack your own beta cells in the pancreas, and it is an autoimmune disease. You get type 1 diabetes. Beta cells in the pancreas produce insulin.

Early exposure to cow's milk can increase the risk of diabetes in the child by about 1.5 times (Cow's Milk Exposure and Type I Diabetes Mellitus: A critical overview of the clinical literature doi.org/10.2337/diacare.17.1.13). Diabetes also does not occur in rodents that are prone to diabetes, and there was no cow's milk in the first two to three months of life, which indicates that the cow's milk protein can activate the disease (New England Journal of Medicine, 1992; 327 (5): 302-307). This information was available for a long time, but people just did not want to believe it. In New Zealand, there was medical controversy about this, and to this day, many farmers have moved on to their own initiative to grow cows that give A2 milk. Researchers from London and Rome announced that they were discovered by examining 47 patients with recently developing insulin-dependent diabetes mellitus (IDDM) and found that in 51% of their immune cells they grew and multiplied when they were exposed to beta-casein protein, from cow's milk. Only 2.7% of healthy people in the control group had immune cells that responded to cow's milk protein. Protein is a problem. There is no animal today in the world, which naturally continues to consume milk to adulthood. Cats do drink milk when given by humans. Every veterinary association in the world if asked would say: "Do not feed your cat with milk, because it causes kidney failure." In cat's blood in urine and red color of urine occurs after consuming more substantial amounts of milk.

And what about lactose tolerance. Lactase is an enzyme that allows the organism to digest milk sugar, and that sugar is lactose. By now we have been looking at the protein, and now we are going to look at the sugar. Danes are only 2% lactose intolerant. Let's explain what exactly this means. All mammals after weaning are lactase deficient. They do not have contact with the milk later in life. The reaction of any organism that do not need to use the sugar lactose in adulthood is to deactivate the enzyme lactase so that the enzyme lactase is deactivated at the level of the genes. Except for the Europeans, which forced their bodies for thousands of years to consume it. Thus, Danes today are only 2% non-tolerant, Finland 18%, Israeli Jews 58%, African Americans 70%, Ashkenazi Jews 78%, Arabs 78%, Eskimos 80%, Taiwanese 85%, Greek Cypriots 85%, Japanese 85%, Thailand 90%, Filipinos 90%, African Blacks over 90%. WHO has put those numbers up, saying that it is around 95% to 100% for African Blacks. For American Indians 90 to 100, for Asians 90 to 95, for Mediterranean 60 to 75 and North Americans 10 to 15 and white Europeans 5 to 10 percent. India is good example of this. In South India intolerance is about 66.6% but in Northern India for example in New Delhi the intolerance is much lower 27.4% (Lactose intolerance in North and South Indians. Am J Clin Nutr. 1981 May;34(5):943-6). The lower incidence in the North Indian subjects is due to the fact that they are descendants of the Aryans from Europe and the same situation can be seen in parts of Iran and in all of the Ancient Persian tribes in Central Asia and Asia Minor. Iran is just Middle Persian word for Aryan, but it includes all of the people outside of the country that is named Iran (from the Avestan term airyanəm vaējah for homeland of Arians to include all of the Persian Arian tribes outside of Iran known as old Iranian term aryānām xšaθra, approximately "expanse of the Aryans", i.e. Iranians). Haplogroup R1a is found for example in Russia (65%), Poland (57.5%) but not in Germany (only in eastern parts around 20% that were initially settled by Slavic tribes but then conquered and assimilated under Charlemagne in Early Middle Ages). Then also the highest frequency of R1a in the world beside European part of Russia is reached in a cluster around Tajikistan, Kyrgyzstan and northern Afghanistan (65%). These people at least genetically and some of them also historically today consider themselves as Iranian tribes. Then Northern India is 50%. The highest cluster in the world in not found in European Slavic tribes but actually within Brahmins (highest caste in Hinduism and they do not like to mix with other lower casts) belonging to R1a1 haplogroup 70%. Dravidian-speaking South (Tamil Nadu, Kerala, Karnataka, Andhra Pradesh) and from Bengal eastward have 22% of R1a1 and as a consequence 66% of them are lactose intolerant. This might be strange to you that Indo-European languages only survived in Slavic Russia and Iran or in the southern part of Central Asia, in places like Afghanistan, Tajikistan, or some parts of Turkmenistan? Why don't the Kyrgyzs, Uzbeks, Kazakhs or Uyghurs or the modern Pontic-Caspian steppe people (Bashkirs, Chuvashs, Crimean Tatars, Nogais) speak Indo-European dialects? Genetically these people do mostly carry Indo-European R1a, and to a lesser extent also R1b, lineages. The explanation is that Turkic languages replaced the Iranian tongues of Central Asia between the 4th and 11th century CE. Spread started with the Hunnic migrations westward through the Eurasian steppe and all the way to Europe. The Huns were the descendants of the Xiongnu a hybrid Eurasian people 2,000 years ago, with mixed European and North-East Asian Y-DNA and mtDNA (Mongolian lineages). I already analyzed in first part of the series when the first lactose tolerance emerged. Scientific research confirmed in different ancient European genome studies that the hunter-gatherers in Europe could not digest lactose in milk at 8000 years ago. The first Europeans that domesticated wild animals were also unable to consume milk. The settlers who came from the Near East about 7800 years ago also couldn't. The Yamnaya pastoralists who came to Europe from the eastern steppes around 4800 years ago also couldn't. It was not until about 2300 BC about 4300 years ago, in the Early Bronze Age, that lactose tolerance swept through Europe and then spread eastward with migrations from Eastern Europe. Only descendants of first European farmers from Early Bronze Age can tolerate lactose, the rest of the human population cannot. It is not their food.

Let me show you how sugar lactose is metabolized. We have enzyme lactase that breaks sugar lactose on dextrose and sugar named galactose. It is important for a baby because baby metabolism is not fast enough yet that it only gets half as glucose and the other half as galactose. However, galactose cannot be used until it is digested to glucose. There is an enzyme called beta-galactosidase that changes galactose to the glucose that we need. However, since no animal needs this enzyme after weaning this enzyme is deactivated forever. Forever and ever for whites also. Everyone, every human on the planet earth if it is grown adult has galactosidase deficiency. All of you who are reading this now have a deficiency of beta-galactosidase. This means that if you consume sugar from milk meaning lactose, if you are white, you are from Europe, you can use it, you have lactase. Lactase metabolizers lactose and you will get glucose and beside it also a galactose. Glucose will be used normally. And with galactose, what are you going to do? You cannot use it so where does galactose go? What our body is to do with galactose? Some of it gets ejected outside thru the skin. Some end up in the eyes and are stored in the cornea. Elderly cataracts come from galactose. Adults who consume large amounts of milk, who have high lactase activity, often suffer from galactose, accumulation of galactitol in the eye lobe and have a high likelihood of elderly cataracts. (Postgraduate Medicine 1994; 95 (1): 115). Not only that, it is stored in the body in other places as well. Women are accumulating around the ovaries, and it is associated with cancer of the ovaries and infertility also. One in four couples goes to infertility treatments in European countries where milk is consumed. All of them are extremely well-fed. In African countries, where they do not use milk, they have no problems with infertility. It is unknown as a disease.

Here's the famous Daniel W. Cramer Harvard Medical School study here (Dairy foods and nutrients in relation to risk of ovarian cancer and major histological subtypes doi: [10.1002/ijc.27701]). Cramer saw a link between the consumption of galactose and the increased risk of ovarian cancer. Considering that lactose intolerant women are likely to consume less lactose, and they list the number of studies. They concluded that: "This finding suggests that decreased lactose intake early in life may reduce ovarian cancer risk although further studies are needed to confirm this finding." Many studies would suggest that this sugar may affect fertility. His team compared the published data from 36 countries regarding the fertility rate, milk consumption per capita, and hypolactasia. They now published a correlation between high rates of consumption of milk and declining fertility, which begins in women who have just 20-24 years of age. This is published in the American Journal of Epidemiology. For Thai women, for example, who do not consume milk, there is no infertility at the level of statistical significance. The severity of this relationship and the decline in fertility increased with each of the following groups studied, with age increasing in each of the following groups. In Thailand for example, where 98% of adults are lactose intolerant, the average fertility among women aged 35-39 years was only 26% lower than the maximum rate for ages 25-29 years. In Australia and the UK, where lactose intolerance affects only 5% of adult people the fertility rates for 35-39 years old are full 82% below the maximum rate for ages 25-29 years.

What will happen when an individual that is not tolerant of lactose drinks milk? If Africans consumed milk that do not have lactase enzyme, what would happen? It will cause lactose to be broken down by bacteria in the intestines. When lactose starts to split, this increases osmotic pressure, fluid flows into the intestines, and they get diarrhea. White people do not have lactose problems, so they do not get diarrhea, but still have a massive problem with the casein, and galactose and saturated fat and in recent years, antibiotics and hormones and other toxins and pesticides found in milk. Many babies who drink cow's milk will experience obstipation interventions where there is a special tool that physically removes excrement outside because of the impossibility of discharge. They usually didn't know what was the cause of children constipation that in some cases prolong to adulthood. They prescribed the usual therapy of high fiber intake and laxative drugs. However, this study solved the mystery (Intolerance of cow's milk and chronic constipation in children. N Engl J Med. 1998 Oct 15;339(16):1100-4). They took 65 children with chronic constipation, and all of them were treated with laxatives. They designed the study and gave them soy milk and cow's milk and then switch them around. The ones on soy started to drink the cow's milk, and the one drinking cow mils started to drink soy. In 44 out of 65 children 68% constipation resolved when they were on the soy milk. None of the children drinking regular cow's milk had any positive response. Some of the children have severe lesions, and anal fissures and all of that was cured when they were off the cow's milk and then reappeared in days after they were back on the cow's milk. Changing up cow's milk can also help to cure anal fissures in adults also. This is nothing new. Studies around the world were able to cure constipation in children to the number of about 80% just by giving up the milk. Why 80 or 68 percent? Because giving up on milk does not mean giving up on all dairy protein. Some of the children still might consume some milk chocolate or eat ice-cream or something containing powder milk and not even be aware of it. When they design a study in 2003 that controlled for all milk protein the constipation cure rate in children was, can you guess? It was a 100 percent cure rate (Does Milk Cause Constipation? A Crossover Dietary Trial doi.org/10.3390/nu5010253). All participants in this study experienced resolution. On another hand in lactose intolerant baby's diarrhea occurs.

After World War 2 US had a big stockpile of powdered milk that they had to dispose of somehow. Instead, they decided that because there is a "protein gap" they send that powder milk to Africa as humanitarian aid. Many already malnourished children and babies got diarrhea from it. African countries that got milk powder sent as humanitarian aid experienced an increase in mortality especially in small children who were already at the level of severe malnutrition. They then drank milk concentrate, which in it contains lactose itself, got terrible diarrhea and died. They were practically killed by poison, sent from the US under the UN. This happened also due to the degree of non-education in poor African populations that were not familiar with the problem of intolerance to dairy sugar. Now UN does not send any form of milk as humanitarian aid, ever. In Africa when they learned the lesson they used the powder as a paint to paint their sheds into white. This topic is serious.

Or how about this. The leukemia virus is present in 60% of milk on the market. The antibodies of leukemia virus in cattle (BLV) are present in 59% of newborn test calves. (Canadian J of Comparative Medicine 1979; 43 (2): 173-179). Now, this is bovine not human leukemia-causing virus. However, there can be a mutation that allows the virus to cross species. That is how we can get new strains of flu viruses from birds for example that we do not have immune system defense and everyone gets scared when you say a bird flu virus. Same thing with leukemia or any other virus. Just remember the HIV for instance.

Human T cell leukemia viruses can be transmitted from humans to animals and from animals to humans. This result suggests that the infection in the milk of a mother she transmits to her baby is entirely possible. And also the ability to get cattle leukemia virus to mutate from cattle to humans is studied in many studies. Statistically, countries using dairy cow products have more leukemia. For example, Iowa (dairy state) has more rates than the national average for human leukemia (Epidemiologic relationships of the bovine population and human leukemia in Iowa doi.org/10.1093/oxfordjournals.aje.a112979). Pennsylvania veterinarians were able to cultivate BLV in human cells in a lab. Studies of 1980 showed an increase in human leukemia in areas with high rates of leukemia in cattle (Science, 1981; 213 (4511): 1014-1016). Do you think this is a small problem? About 86% of the population in the U.S. have bovine leukemia virus antibodies detected, and by 1995 they knew that this virus works on humans as well. This study in 2003 with much better detection equipment then confirmed results from the 1980s that we are exposed. It showed the same thing (Humans have antibodies reactive with Bovine leukemia virus. AIDS Res Hum Retroviruses. 2003 Dec;19(12):1105-13). And this is all caused by the original problem, and that is that the virus makes the cows produce more milk. What cows will the farmer keep, the one that produces more milk or the one that produces less? Cows infected with BLV have significantly higher production than their blood donor, who are not infected with BLV. This means that much more milk is produced with BLV than previously estimated (Proceedings of the National Academy of Sciences of the United States of America, 1989; 86 (3): 993-996). These data confirm the presence of BLV in milk and identify the potential for lactogenic (dairy) transmission of the virus (American Journal of Veterinary Research, 1995; 56 (4): 445-449). Remember these are all top scientific journals and research, not nonsense, and other diseases could also be transmitted through milk. Several conditions such as tuberculosis, brucellosis, diphtheria, Scarlet fever, Q-fever, and gastroenteritis are transmitted through dairy products. Milk is an excellent transporter of infections because its fat content protects pathogens from gastric acid and since fat in milk has a relatively short gastric transient time.

Due to this milk property, pasteurization and sterilization are obligatory by law. However, these methods do not only destroy all the toxins and all forms of pathogens in milk. Pasteurization does kill all of the bacteria but also some of the vital enzymes (catalase, peroxidase, phosphatase) and vitamins. It also extends its durability for commercial use in order to the prolong the fresh appearance of the milk and that ensures that the bacteria would not develop further in it. However, when enzymes such as phosphate are destroyed, milk loses nutritional value. Namely, phosphatases serve to break the food in our organism so that cells can assimilate mineral salts from it that are in the form of phytate. Unfortunately, the human organism does not have adequate levels of these phosphatase enzymes at all, as rats do. Lack of these enzymes will cause a lowering of the absorption of minerals that are in the form of phytates. Phytic acid acts as an anti-nutritive agent by blocking the absorption of minerals such as Fe, Zn, and Ca. A phosphatase is found only in raw milk and whole grains of cereals. If pasteurization of milk were not to be carried out, it would have to be clean and produced under far better hygienic conditions, or its poor condition would be visible by visible clumping before reaching the customer. Pasteurization destroys the phosphatase enzyme. And this is a sure mark that the milk is pasteurized. The protein value (amino acid composition) is reduced by 17%. From the metabolic data, it is concluded that the heat is damaging to lysine and probably histidine and other amino acids, vitamin A is destroyed, vitamins D, E, K are unchanged, vitamin B complex is destroyed 38%, vitamin C is destroyed. Concerning calcium itself, its utilization has been significantly reduced.

So what is so good about the milk? What about the casein from milk (especially A1 beta-casein)? What about milk sugar (lactose)? What about milk fat? And what about calcium and other minerals and vitamins after the pasteurization? So far, we have not considered the impact of toxins, hormones, antibiotics, and other substances. Bovine somatotropin or BGH since 1994 was used in the production of cattle meat and was obtained by reconstitution DNA technology. Recombinant bovine growth hormone (rBGH), or growth hormone. Monsanto is the first company to develop technology, and it advertised him as a Savior. The presence of rBGH in the cow stimulates the production of the second hormone Insulin-Like Growth Factor-1, or IGF-1. IGF-1 is the one that is directly responsible of increasing milk production. IGF-1 naturally occurs both in cows and in humans. IGF-1 is not destroyed during pasteurization nor when digesting. It is interesting that it has the same molecular composition for both cows and humans. This is the only hormone known to have the same composition in two different species in nature, and is therefore considered to be biologically active in humans, associated with cancer breast, prostate, and colon, in addition to another set of disorders such as premature puberty in children. Dr. Frank M. Biro, head of the Department of Adolescent Medicine at the Cincinnati Children's Hospital Center and his colleagues, found that 15% of

Latino-American girls, more than 10% white woman and 25% of Afro-American women started puberty as early as seven years old. The research was conducted among 1,238 children aged 6 to 8 years from various cities in the United States. Posilac (recombinant DNA-derived bovine somatotropin) is banned in Canada, Australia, New Zealand, Japan, and the EU countries. A healthy cow supplemented with Posilac® produces an average of 10 more pounds of milk per day. The question is, if there is apparent disagreement between different countries, then the picture looks like as the science is the problem. One country scientist finds something harmless to use, and then the scientists from another country consider it to be an illegal poison. In the book Milk: The Deadly Poison, author Robert Cohen has been researching billions of dollars dairy and pharmaceutical industries were spent on influencing the FDA and the Congress as well as for the impact on the scientific and medical establishment and a whole series of court processes against the dairy industry. Milk today is a non-replaceable food product for a simple reason because its rejection from human use would mean the economic problem of global proportions in a world where more than a billion people live below the poverty line. The diet itself is just as an economic and political issue as the medicine and health. Chronic illnesses are the most stable source of income at the level of the military industrial complex or in the fields of oil production. Tendencies in the food industry today are going to the highest possible volume of production in order to achieve high profits, which is economically justified. More of the research goes to the genetically modified crops, and in markets that are still in development, such as China, India, and countries of the third world where high-level malnutrition is present. Demand for food products and expectations that food demand will continue to grow in the near future is all we need to know when we look at the business model of food production. What can be expected is that the prices of industrial produced food will remain on the same level, the quality of food will decrease, and genetically modified foods will be increasingly used, both in humans and in fodder.

What is known to associated with dairy product use is chronic fatigue, headaches, hyperactivity (ADD, ADHD), allergy and congestion, asthma and respiratory problems, early arteriosclerosis from oxidized cholesterol and cardiac arterial disease, diabetes type 1, rheumatoid arthritis, multiple sclerosis, decline of the intelligence, pimples, bedwetting, ovarian cancer, cataract, osteoporosis and IGF-1 related diseases. In cow's milk are bacteria, viruses, prions, and antibiotics, hormones, pesticides, and other toxins and heavy metals.

Pimples from all things? Well, acne is an epidemic in western countries. This skin disease affects around 85% of adolescents, but in more natural plant eating communities like Okinawa Islanders or Kitavan Islanders there were no cases

(Evidence for acne-promoting effects of milk and other insulinotropic dairy products. doi: 10.1159/000325580). Not a single one. In rural parts of China and India it is very rare disease so it must be a one more bad reaction coming from the diet. Same people when migrate to the western countries and start to accept the western diet develop acne at the same level. Why is this correlated to milk? Because of the androgenic hormones naturally present in milk and all other dairy products even without additionally added Posilac (somatotropin). These androgenic hormones are stable and cannot be fermented or destroyed by pasteurization. There are there to promote the growth of the newborn calf's. Studies had proved these hormones are in dairy products, and this has a direct effect on the oil-producing glands in human skin. The problem is that if they are androgenic, they also stimulate other things as well. How about premature puberty. These hormones also stimulate cancer growth. Especially hormone-dependent cancers like breast and prostate cancer (Acne, dairy, and cancer: The 5alpha-P link. Dermatoendocrinol. 2009 Jan;1(1):12-6). The 5alpha-P is the androgenic or sex hormone present in milk. And no there is no adding of this hormone by industry. Organic milk has it, and it is naturally present in all dairy products. For instance, back acne is 100% exclusively caused by overconsumption of dairy products. Problem with these dairy sex hormones is that our bodies do not have a natural feedback loop. If you are a bodybuilder and decide to inject steroids, your body will detect that hormone and shut down your own production trying to keep the testosterone in a normal range. However, for 5alpha-P there is no feedback loop, our brain does not detect it and does not decrease the production of any sex hormones both testosterone or its derivate DHT and estrogen. So when you eat excessive dairy, it is like you have just injected yourself with some more DHT and estrogen. In our natural evolution, there was no need to develop receptors in our brain to tell us that we have some more cow milk sex hormones in our body. It is just one more maladaptation. Acne is a cosmetic issue, you can take some Accutane and be done with it, but when you get breast or prostate cancer, then you can die. It all comes in a package. Excessive DHT might give us some acne and increased libido and make us bald, but excessive estrogen is a problem. The real problem of dairy consumption.

In men it will lead to infertility in a woman it would lead to breast cancer. All food of animal origin will have estrogen in it. Cows estrogen work as good as human estrogen. By drinking a 300mg or one glass milk a day a child will increase consumption of estradiol-17β the most potent form of all estrogens for about 10ng. This is 4000 times as potent as environmental exposure to xenoestrogen because of xenoestrogen lower level of potency (Is milk responsible for male reproductive disorders? Med Hypotheses. 2001 Oct;57(4):510-4.). A conclusion of this study was:" Milk and dairy products, are responsible for 60-70% of the estrogens consumed in the western diet. Humans consume milk obtained from heifers in the latter half of pregnancy when the estrogen levels in cows are markedly elevated. The milk that we now consume may be quite unlike that consumed 100 years ago. Modern genetically-improved dairy cows, such as the Holstein, are usually fed a combination of grass and concentrates (grain/protein mixes and various by-products), allowing them to lactate during the latter half of pregnancy, even at 220 days of gestation. We hypothesize that milk is responsible, at least in part, for some male reproductive disorders." When cows are not pregnant the amount of estrogen in milk is around 30pg/ml. However, because of the way the business is run on the farms most of the cows are pregnant, and the levels of estradiol in the pregnant cows are hundreds of times higher. For example, from 220 to 240 days of gestation, the levels of estradiol are at the maximum at 1000pg/ml. From 30 to 1000. On top of that add some 5alpha-P and Posilac. Dairy is associated to lower sperm count and movement and direct testicular damage. It as damaging to testis as cholesterol. Maybe even more. However, who cares about that?

Main marketing scam they use to sell dairy products is that they contain calcium. Numerous factors cause osteoporosis, and lack of dietary calcium is not one of them. Not even that statement that milk is full of calcium if entirely correct. It is not what you eat. It is what you absorb. Only 25% of calcium in cow milk is absorbable by the body after pasteurization, which is due to destroyed enzymes. Human milk, although it contains half the amount of calcium compared to cow's milk, is a better source of calcium because of its high absorption capacity. Even certain plants like poppy seeds or sesame seeds are better sources for the same reason. These are bad news!

Is the situation the same with cheese, yogurt or any other dairy product? What is the real distinction between milk and cheese? A bacterial culture is taken, it is then added to the milk, fermentation takes place and the whey is separated from it. From the solid part, cheese is made. First separation creates soft cheese and in time the old cheese will mature. Why does it mature? Because bacteria culture in the cheese is allowed to develop more. When bacteria have used everything, you get matured cheese. Bacteria will not consume the protein, so there is a lot of casein in it. Bacteria will not consume fat or cholesterol or any other fat molecule. Only sugar (lactose) is eaten, and only part that consist of glucose. Bacteria cannot do much with galactose either so cheese contains much of galactose too. So kefir, yogurt cheeses are the same as milk just without lactose and can be consumed by people sensitive to lactose, but they are still full of galactose (ovarian cancer, cataract) and fat and casein. Dairy products are very acid forming for the body. The amount of acid formed by food per mEq / 100g edible meat meal and meat products is 9.5, cheese, small protein content (<15%)

is 8, for cheese with high protein content (> 15%) is 23.6, vegetables -2.8, fruit and fruit juices -3.1. What does the organism do with so much acid in the body I already explained in the previous chapter. Experiments were performed on rats that were exclusively fed by casein. The consequence was that their urine was very acidic.

Now, let's repeat all this knowledge. We absorb only 25% of calcium from pasteurized milk and all other pasteurized milk products. It is filled with cholesterol. In experiments on rabbits, results have been obtained that the casein itself elevates the level of bad cholesterol, even without cholesterol from milk. The following results were obtained: blood cholesterol level (mg/dl), average vegetable protein 67, crude protein 101, pork protein 107, chicken protein 138, beef protein 152, protein from fish 160, protein from whole egg 176, casein from milk 203, protein from skim milk 225. Milk is the second in the list of food products that raise cholesterol. Protein rises cholesterol and a 0% milk fat will not help you. It is worst of them all actually. You will get cholesterol and especially bad cholesterol. The milk is bad for the heart and whole cardiovascular system and for the bones. When you have osteoporosis, doctors will recommend the standard therapy for calcium supplements. You will take more milk and create even more significant problems, and everything is worse and worse.

There is no correlation among milk consumption and reduced risk of osteoporosis. Someone have been spreading lies and myths to fool and trick people (Milk intake and risk of hip fracture in men and women: a meta-analysis of prospective cohort studies. doi: 10.1002/jbmr.279.). When we look at all the studies what we found is actually the opposite. The countries with the greatest milk consumption also have the biggest risk of osteoporosis. Not even during childhood and adolescence milk consumption have no association with bone density. It even seems that it will increase the risk later in life. These studies are so well known and so old, and everything you read here has been known by industry for decades. Everything you believe about milk is the lie. We are just addicted to it because of the taste and morphine effect it has. Do not give your children heroin or in other words milk chocolate and ice-cream. So why is the milk so bad for the bones? Calcium had nothing to do with this. Ok, let settle the "enigma" that everybody knows, but nobody is telling. There is a rare birth defect known as galactosemia. It is a genetic mutation that causes a complete lack of enzymes that are needed to detoxify the galactose. Galactose cannot be turned into glucose and used as energy. Not even bacteria can eat it. It has to be detoxified out. What this birth defect of galactosemia does to the kids is that it causes bone loss even as kids (Skeletal health in adult patients with classic galactosemia. doi: 10.1007/s00198-012-1983-0). Do you know what scientist use in studies to cause premature aging in laboratory animals? Can you guess? They use the same thing galactose. Even in small doses, galactose increases the changes that resemble natural aging. Galactose does not just cause bone loss, because it goes everywhere it causes overall inflammation and brain damage and degeneration also.

When scientist understood that milk has a toxic effect on the body, they did one big study that followed 100,000 man and women for 20 years (Milk intake and risk of mortality and fractures in women and men: cohort studies. doi: 10.1136/bmj.g6015). This was cohort study done in central Sweden. The conclusion was: "For every glass of milk, the adjusted hazard ratio of all-cause mortality was 1.15 in women and 1.03 in men. High milk intake was associated with higher mortality in one cohort of women and in another cohort of men, and with higher fracture incidence in women." Milk drinking was associated with inflammation, cancer, bone loss, heart disease. Three glasses of milk a day had raised the total mortality association to be unbelievable 1.93. That means that you have doubled your chances of dying if you drink three glasses of milk a day or 680 grams a day. To conclude the more milk, the more death and bone fractures. That means that milk is a poison like any other poison. The association with mortality was little lower for other milk products like kefir or yogurt or cheese, and that goes along with galactose theory very well. Bacteria that ferment lactose to create yogurt or cheese can partially lower the galactose content. Not completely just partially.

You can try to drink low-fat lactose-free milk, but then you are just consuming milk protein that is bad just by itself. Did you know that dietary food item most associated with Parkinson disease is milk consumption? In all the studies ever done, the association with milk was absolute. At first, the scientist did not know what to think about it. They thought it is some neurotoxin that must be present in milk like organochlorine residues or pesticides. However, if pesticides or organochlorine residues or whatever other toxin is a cause of Parkinson disease, there is no logical explanation why there is no correlation between other food items that have the same toxins and the Parkinson's. Or for example, pesticides build up in fat, but the link between skim milk and Parkinson's is as strong as full-fat milk. And then because they were unable to explain the association they said it is reverse causation. Parkinson disease causes people to became depressed and depressed people drink more milk. However, then prospective cohort studies still were finding the link between milk and Parkinson excluding reverse causation explanation (Dairy foods intake and risk of Parkinson's disease: a dose-response meta-analysis of prospective cohort studies. doi: 10.1007/s10654-014-9921-4). The linear dose-response relationship showed that PD risk increased by 17% [1.17 (1.06-1.30)] for every 200 g/day increment in milk intake and 13% for every slice of cheese. So again all neurotoxins are found in all dairy product so why does cheese have a lower association. And the only thing that cheese has lower than the milk is guess what. The galactose content. There are other neurodegenerative diseases like Huntington disease that runs in families. In Huntington, the risk is 2-fold increase meaning the early onset is doubled by dairy consumption. In some people, genetic predisposition can be worsened by galactose, and in all people, the negative effect of galactose will increase the risk of all diseases that it has been associated with including bone loss. In people with galactosemia 20% of them develop a severe form of progressive tremor and ataxia. People with galactosemia learn not to consume the stuff, but until they learn that they have the condition they do consume it, and some of them end up with tremor and ataxia. We know that galactose is neurotoxin just like any other neurotoxin that can cause such issues as ataxia that means you cannot voluntary move your body. So why do you give the stuff to your children? Nobody had told you, or you do not care because milk is good and source of protein and calcium and we need it on a daily bases, or we are going to lose our bones and teeth. There is absolutely nothing good in milk. Not even calcium. African women do not get osteoporosis on 350mg of calcium per day, and women in Europe receive osteoporosis at 1400mg per day. We will need to find another source of calcium than our milk. The source from whole plant foods. Green vegetables such as kale are as good as milk regarding calcium content.

African women who eat vegetables and legumes and do not drink milk do not have the problem of osteoporosis. There are studies tested on rats and rabbits, but the velvet monkey is considered a better model for humans. In one study these monkeys are fed on a Western diet in one and the African diet in the second group while they were on the milk they lost calcium significantly. And don't forget infertility. We have already said that women have reduced fertility due to galactose. What about the men? Are they immune? The study on the monkeys was carried out in the next course. They were given everything that the monkeys eat bananas and others and then added a little milk powder. The mobility of their sperm dropped. The percentage of sperm counts dropped by 2/3. While there were abnormalities in the sperm count, and it is normal for everyone to have some in this case there were many. Different defects were obtained, the growth and sperm of spermatozoa were changed entirely. So, fertility falls if you use milk for 2/3 plus reduced mobility plus defects. What about lymphocytes? If you want to help your immune system, reduce milk in the diet (especially if you have HIV and other serious diseases). Cow's milk consumption can weaken the immune function in children and lead to the problem of the return of infections (Circulating immune complexes in infants fed on cow's milk. Nature, 1978 Apr 13;272(5654):632.). The premature introduction of dairy products in food and high consumption of milk in childhood can increase the risk of diabetes in the teenage age in the child (Diet, cow's milk protein antibodies and the risk of IDDM in Finnish children Diabetologia, 1994; 37 (4): 381-387).

Why don't we take a look at what happened to the blood vessels of those monkeys. When only a little milk was added, the first good and the bad cholesterol ratio was diagnosed. In the picture, you have pictures of the main arteries. The first is crystal clear (988), that is for a monkey who ate corn and legumes. All small vessels are open. This second (920) is for the monkey who consumed milk with corn. Closed everywhere plus a plaque.

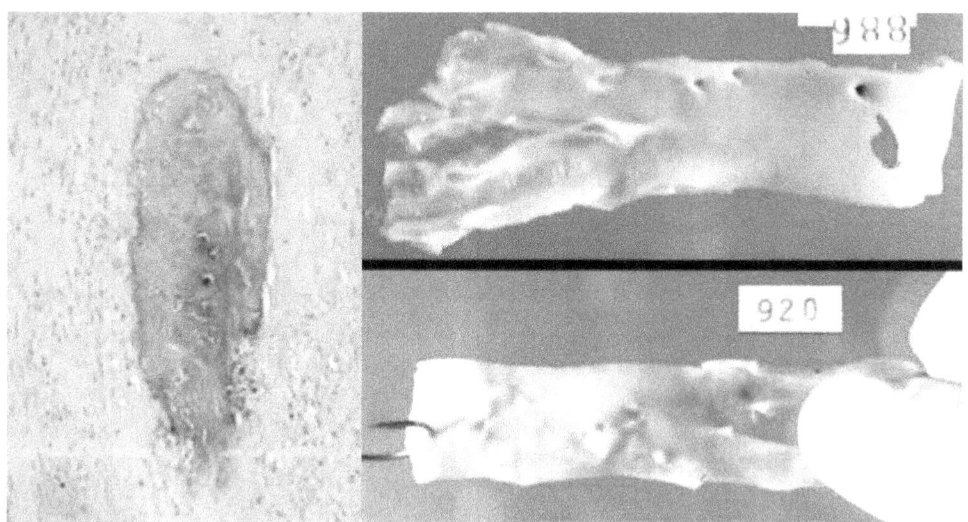

And because they have to drain so much calcium to neutralize the casein, the kidneys cannot get rid of it in time. That is why it sticks to the blood vessels, and you get calcium deposits (picture on the left), and blood vessels become brittle and create the risk of them cracking and blood spilling into the brain (stroke). In this case it is not milk; it can be milk or dairy products or in general any other type of high protein or excess protein diet that will led to calcium deposits on the blood vessels. Also dairy products can play a significant role in the development of allergies due to globular hard to digest protein. Then constipation, difficulty sleeping and migraine pain (Israel Journal of Medical Sciences, 1983; 19 (9): 806-809; Pediatrics, 1989; 84 (4): 595-603).

Now let's analyze diabetes causing by molecular mimicry of A1 beta casein in milk. Beta-casein is about 30% of the protein in cow's milk. Beta-casein is present as one or two genetic variants; A1 or A2. Most cow's milk contains a combination of A1 and A2 beta-casein. However, the milk that contains only the A2 type without A1 beta-casein is available in some countries. Epidemiological evidence suggests that A1 beta-casein is possible risk factor in the development of type 1 diabetes in children and heart illnesses in adults. The second variant, A2 beta-casein, is not associated with these diseases. The established relationship of this link between A1 beta-casein and type 1 diabetes, and heart disease is 0.982 and 0.76. This is a very significant level if compared with other epidemiological reasons for these conditions, such as smoking and mortality from lung cancer r = 0.73 or the likelihood of people in the 1960s to develop heart conditions ten years later where r = 0.85. The difference between A1 and A2 beta-casein is present because of single amino acid substitution at 67 line of amino acids of 209 that they have in the chain. A1 beta-casein in cow's milk is different from all other mammals, which exclusively have A2 type including A2 cattle from Europe or India, Africa, as Buffalo. It is the same with other mammals and the same with human milk. Almost all cattle of the A1 type are related to cows of European origin for the subspecies of the original species of this mutation Bos Taurus. It is a result of a genetic mutation in cows in Europe that happened about 8,000 years ago. Today, A1 cows are breed in Europe and America, A2 species are breed in New Zeeland. Holstein species have A1 and A2 beta-casein in almost equal amounts. The Jersey species typically has a little more than A2 but is also considered as a mixed species. Jersey cows carry also a beta-casein that has proven to give more BCM7. Because of poor histidine (amino acid) attachment, A1 beta-casein breaks down into peptides of 7 amino acids in chain called beta casomorphin 7 (BCM7) when consumed. BCM7 is problematic because it is opiate at the same level as narcotics like morphine and has similar effects. It is also an oxidant that is known to be detrimental to low-density lipoproteins (LDL). Because the links between 7 amino acids that make it are extremely strong, it is resistant to further degradation. When BCM7 enter the bloodstream, various problems arise.

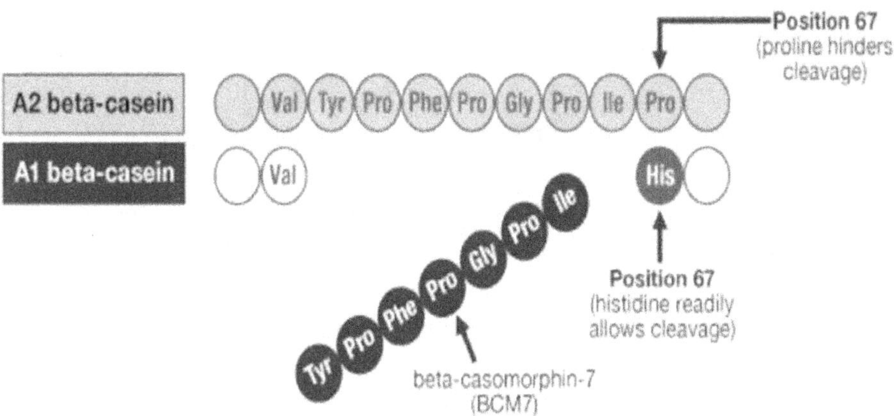

However, the BCM7 is too large to be absorbed by a healthy coat in the intestine, which means that the health problem associated with A1 beta-casein is more likely to affect people with damaged digestive health or from diseases such as celiac disease or gastrointestinal disease. If you have leaky gut, then you and your child can give yourself diabetes if you consume milk and dairy products as an autoimmune disease. Individuals having any of the prevailing conditions are more suitable for excess of BCM7 in bloodstream. In babies that naturally have increased intestinal permeability in order to improve the absorption of nutrients, there is a higher risk also. Once it enters the bloodstream, BCM7 can easily break through the blood-brain barrier and enter into the brain, where the connection to the receptors causes the symptoms of autism and schizophrenia. This claim was initiated by research that was disseminated on rats, where rats showed similar tendencies in behavior and sympathy as autism and schizophrenia after BCM7 injection. The association of these effects was also confirmed by the ability to reverse the state and changes in opioid antagonistic naloxone behavior. To add to that, it has long been recognized that opiates have an effect on the immune function, which is the possible reason why A1 beta-casein and BCM7 are associated with autoimmune diseases. In the case of cardiac diseases, additional studies have uncovered the mechanism by which the A1 beta-casein will develop. BCM7 oxidizes LDL that transports cholesterol from the liver to the tissue. This is important because the oxidized LDL increases the risk of heart disease as a result of increased artery incidence and as a consequence Increased plaque accumulation.

As for type 1 diabetes, it is classified as an autoimmune disease that occurs due to an immune system assault on cells that produce insulin in the pancreas. And it is not genetic as you might lead to believe by conventional medicine. Genetic predisposition plays a role but to prove the fact that it is just one more maladaptation we can look at identical twins. Concordance of diabetes type 1 in identical twins is only 50 %. Meaning one gets it one not. If it is genetic and environment does not play a role that would not happen. It is something we ate or to be precise mother ate or give their baby's that causes them to develop this autoimmune disease. In Japan diabetes type 1 is 18 times lower than in the US, but when Japanese migrate to the America and star to adopt the western diet, they develop the same rate of diabetes as Americans have. Some countries have 100 of times the less diabetes type 1 rates than others depending mostly on the diet the population eats. Type one diabetes started to rise after World War 2 as same as other diseases, so it is not genetics. It is maladaptation, and we now know what is causing it. In 1999 scholar in Germany discovered what that there is a correlation between type 1 diabetes and the level of antibodies to A1 beta-casein. It is believed that these antibodies are, in fact, based on the amino acid sequence of the problematic opioid BCM7, which is derived from A1 beta-casein. Because the sequence has similarities with the protein structure of the cells that produce insulin in the pancreas, the antibodies attack the pancreas together with the BCM7 peptides. In this study, every single child had significant levels of A1 beta casein antibodies in their blood but not of antibodies to other milk proteins (A bovine albumin peptide as a possible trigger of insulin-dependent diabetes mellitus. N Engl J Med. 1992 Jul 30;327(5):302-7). The conclusion was: "Patients with insulin-dependent diabetes mellitus have immunity to cows milk albumin, with antibodies to an albumin peptide that is capable of reacting with a beta-cell-specific surface protein. Such antibodies could participate in the development of islet dysfunction."

Also, there are opiates that cross the blood-brain barrier. Because BCM7 opiates should not be present at all and represent a form of unnatural mutation in cattle it should not be the great surprise in the relationship between A1 beta-casein and the casein in general to association with autism also. BCM 7 obtained from A1 beta-casein and gluteomorphin derived from gluten are both opiates that can be associated with these symptoms. Because of this, a huge number of children with autism show significant improvements if they avoid gluten and casein. The relationship between autism and opiates is nothing new. In 1979, Jaak Panksepp, a scientist, suggested that connection. In 2000, a team of researchers led by Robert Cade reviewed the existing evidence linking the casein and gluten opiates with autism and schizophrenia. They collected new data from 150 autistic children, 120 schizophrenia adults, 43 normal children and 76 normal adults. Autistic children and schizophrenia adults showed a constant elevated abnormal value of casomorphin and gluteomorphin opioid peptides obtained from beta-casein and gluten. Actually all adults show elevated levels of this morphine opioid substance after consumption of milk or yogurt, even the adult that do not have inflammation in the gut at least for 8 hours after consumption (Casein peptide release and passage to the blood in humans during digestion of milk or yogurt. Biochimie. 1998 Feb;80(2):155-65.). The theory goes something like this. You have a genetic predisposition for diseases such as autism or schizophrenia. This is the so-called "opioid excess" theory. So you have a genetic predisposition and then have some early exposure to environmental stressors that damage your gut or you are just a regular baby that naturally has leaky gut. Then comes the milk or dairy products with all of the casomorphins leaking into the blood in excess then into the brain triggering disease to form. These opioids are thought that could play one of the roles in the development of autism and other neurological disorders. The problem with this casomorphins is also that when you examine the blood-brain barrier of autism patients, their blood-brain barrier seams weaker too. In a normal individual, there are going to be some of the sedative effects but in someone with leaky gut and the leaky blood-brain barrier it is going to have a much stronger effect, and if that person has genetic predisposition or sensitivity to it then the real disease can form. By so-called "opioid excess" theory anyway. Of the seventy autistic children placed on a gluten-free and casein-free diet, 81% showed significant improvements over a period of 3 months, and more than a third of those who did not recover were still high in opioid peptides, indicating that they did not keep the child diet. Although only 40% of adults have improved, it is believed that many of them have not been using the diet for long enough to provide their body with the ability to eliminate existing BCM7 molecules in the brain that can last for more than a year. In 1999, Zhongjie Sun and Robert Cade injected BCM7 opioid derivatives from A1 beta-casein into rats to determine if it enters the brain. They found out that it will enter to the various areas of the brain that were previously proven to be associated with autism and schizophrenia. As a consequence, it was reasoned that the BCM7 could break through a blood-brain barrier, and hit parts of the brain that are susceptible to those effected by autism and schizophrenia. In the same year, they conducted a similar experiment and found that rats injected with BCM7 exhibited several significant symptoms for autism and schizophrenia such as intolerance, reduced pain sensitivity, and lack of response to external stimuli. In 2003, Sun and Cade continued their research and discovered are that gluteomorphin opioid derived from gluten affects only three regions of the brain while BCM7 opioid was derived from A1 beta-casein affected 45 regions. This not only proved that BCM7 comes to the brain much more easily but it is also a much larger factor in the development of autism and schizophrenia. Are these studies going to lead to more understanding or better treatment of these individuals I do not know. There could be individuals with a genetic predisposition to these diseases that these molecular mimicry proteins only aggravate. I don't know. Science still doing research but it is a slow process and who will have the interest to finance these studies. It will take some time.

A1 or A2 milk had become the big political issue in Australia and New Zeeland at one point. It ended with obligatory labeling of the milk and all dairy products. In Australia, you cannot buy a bottle of milk or any other dairy product without the visible label that shows does the milk contain A1 or A2 form of protein. Why are these opioids in the milk in the first place? For normal human baby or calf, they are there to create a craving to get them addicted in the same way that regular drug addicts are. In this case, the addiction is going to trigger the baby's craving for opiates and then the baby is going to get all the nutrition from milk that it needs to grow. It is all as it should be but now we have switched species. Just like the protein amino acid profile of human and cow milk is not the same the profile of these casomorphins are also not the same. In this study (Beta-casomorphins-7 in infants on different type of feeding and different levels of psychomotor development. doi: 10.1016/j.peptides.2009.06.025.) the baby's fed on cow's milk with a higher level of bovine casomorphins seams to suffer from psychomotor delay but exactly reverse was found for human casomorphins. Human casomorphins are weaker and it seems that they actually help the brain of humans. The conclusion of the study was: "The highest basal irHCM (human casomorphins) was observed in breast-fed infants with normal psychomotor development and muscle tone. In contrast, elevated basal irBCM (cattle casomorphins) was found in formula-fed infants showing a delay in psychomotor development and heightened muscle tone. Among formula-fed infants with normal development, the rate of this parameter directly correlated to basal irBCM. The data indicate that breastfeeding has an advantage over artificial feeding for infant development during the first year of life and support the hypothesis for the deterioration of bovine casomorphin elimination as a risk factor for delay in psychomotor development and other diseases such as autism." Structure of casein in human and cow milk are significantly different matching only by 47%, and especially if we have mutated A1 casein in the mix, then we have a situation that can trigger diabetes type 1 in the baby. Bovine casomorphin is much stronger than human one, and it is almost at the level of morphine in its effect (Epigenetic effects of casein-derived opioid peptides in SH-SY5Y human neuroblastoma cells. doi: 10.1186/s12986-015-0050-1.). Cow's casomorphins bind tighter to the serotonin receptors in the brain then human one does. Also, opioid casomorphins were produced by both A1 and A2 milk with no difference in potency (Identification of bioactive peptides and quantification of β-casomorphin-7 from bovine β-casein A1, A2 and I after ex vivo gastrointestinal digestion doi.org/10.1016/j.idairyj.2017.03.008). Also, there is much more casein in general in cow's milk, 15 times more to be precise than in human's milk. Twenty-one peptides and eight from beta-casein were found in cow milk, and only five peptides with only one from beta-casein were found in human milk.

One thing I found people who want to change their diet have the hardest time getting rid of is cheese and dairy. The meat they can do, but cheese is hard. People who eat a vegetarian diet for a moral reasons eventually don't have the real and full health benefits. They just substitute one animal protein like meat for another like eggs and dairy. Same toxins, hormones, inflammation effects. Same IGF-1 level same everything. If you want to have health benefits, you must treat the milk and eggs the same way as you treat meat. As a survival food that is toxic to the body that we can tolerate in small amounts if we do not want to have all of the diseases of affluence. Giving up meat to eat ice-cream all day is not going to do much for your health. Except drugging your brain with casomorphins and exposing you to risk of cancer and diabetes.